HEALING SYNDROME O

HEALING SYNDROME O

A Strategic Guide to Fertility, Polycystic Ovaries, and Insulin Imbalance

RONALD F. FEINBERG, M.D., PH.D.

FERTILITY SPECIALIST, REPRODUCTIVE ASSOCIATES OF DELAWARE

AVERY

a member of Penguin Group (USA) Inc.

New York

Neither the publisher nor the author is engaged in rendering professional advice or services to the individual reader. The ideas, procedures, and suggestions contained in this book are not intended as a substitute for consulting with your physician. All matters regarding health require medical supervision. Neither the author nor the publisher shall be liable or responsible for any loss, injury, or damage allegedly arising from any information or suggestion in this book. The opinions expressed in this book represent the personal views of the author and not of the publisher.

While the author has made every effort to provide accurate telephone numbers and Internet addresses at the time of publication, neither the publisher nor the author assumes any responsibility for errors or for changes that occur after publication.

Most Avery books are available at special quantity discounts for bulk purchase for sales promotions, premiums, fund-raising, and educational needs. Special books or book excerpts also can be created to fit specific needs. For details, write Penguin Group (USA) Inc. Special Markets, 375 Hudson Street, New York, NY 10014.

AVERY

a member of
Penguin Group (USA) Inc.
375 Hudson Street
New York, NY 10014
www.penguin.com

Library of Congress Cataloging-in-Publication Data

Feinberg, Ronald F.
Healing syndrome O : a strategic guide to fertility, polycystic ovaries, and insulin imbalance / Ronald F. Feinberg.
p. cm.
Includes index.
ISBN 1-58333-167-0
1. Stein-Leventhal syndrome. 2. Fertility. 3. Diabetes—Complications.
4. Healing. I. Title.
RG480.S7F456   2004   2004041094
618.1'1—dc22

Printed in the United States of America
3   5   7   9   10   8   6   4   2

This book is printed on acid-free paper. ∞

To my wife, Robin, my daughters, Jennifer and Jacqueline,
and my son, Michael:
Thanks for letting Dad be a doctor and a writer

To all my patients:
Thanks for letting me learn, so I could learn how to help

ACKNOWLEDGMENTS

Many different people helped lay the foundation for *Healing Syndrome O,* in particular the patients I have had the honor of caring for over the past twenty years as a physician. I continue to learn from my patients, as well as from many talented mentors in the specialities of obstetrics, gynecology, and reproductive endocrinology and infertility. In particular, I thank Drs. Sam Thatcher, Fred Naftolin, Alan DeCherney, Luigi Mastroianni, Steve Sondheimer, and Luis Blasco for their perseverance in trying to educate me. Other colleagues who have been vital to my research and thinking processes along the way include Drs. Harvey Kliman, Barbara McGuirk, Ira Studin, Ricardo Loret de Mola, Federico Monzon, Rhonda Karter, Tsai Wang, Steven Sawin, Peter Van Deerlin, Mark Perloe, Richard Legro, Michael Tucker, Charles Lockwood, and Jerome Strauss.

A special thank-you goes to my physician partner at Reproductive Associates of Delaware, Dr. Barbara McGuirk. Her special dedication to her patients and work has been inspirational, and we share many important philosophies of quality care. We couldn't provide that care without the hard work of many wonderful clinical, lab, and administrative staff members at Reproductive Associates.

I am especially grateful to all the terrific people I have gotten to know at the Polycystic Ovarian Syndrome Association, PCOStrategies, Delaware Valley RESOLVE, and the American Infertility Association. Thank you for your diligence, volunteer spirit, and support of the Syndrome O concept. To one person in particular, Lesa Childers, who knows this project happened at a turtle's pace—thank you for being such an understanding coach.

On the literary side, I appreciate the investment that Avery has been willing to make in *Healing Syndrome O,* and a special note of thanks to the people who helped bring this project to fruition—Eileen Bertelli, Amy Brosey, Amy Tecklenburg, Laura Shepherd, and Rebecca Behan. Outstanding editorial assistance and manuscript review was provided by Pamela Liflander. I'd also like to acknowledge Gareth Esersky, of the Carol Mann Agency, for believing in Syndrome O and the new author who conceptualized it.

Ronald F. Feinberg

CONTENTS

Several years ago, at the age of twenty-eight, I was diagnosed with something called *Polycystic Ovarian Syndrome* (PCOS). My doctor explained to me that symptoms for the disease varied wildly from woman to woman, and could include infertility, irregular menses, excessive hair growth, obesity, and acne. It can also increase a woman's risk for diabetes. But after learning about this array of possible symptoms, I was left wondering what this foreign-sounding disease was going to mean to me.

Six years later, while speaking at the annual conference sponsored by the Polycystic Ovarian Syndrome Association, I related my personal struggle to understand and cope with this disease. While 5 to 10 percent of American women of reproductive age are affected by PCOS, there was an astonishing lack of information available to the public regarding the disease—there were no books, Web sites, or magazine articles to turn to for information or compassion. There were no medications approved for the treatment of PCOS, and the treatment protocols in the medical community varied greatly.

Fortunately for me, my diagnosis came during the Internet age. While I couldn't log on to find PCOS education Web sites, I could connect with other women who were sharing my experiences with the disease—women who had been walking this road longer than I had, and who could help me understand what it meant to live with PCOS.

But some of my frustrations remained. PCOS had been "on the books" for more than seventy years at the time of my diagnosis, but there were still no resources available to women with this disorder that often robs them of their womanhood. That day at the PCOS conference, I was speaking in order to call for an increase in the awareness of PCOS, and I believed that to achieve part of that goal, a new name needed to be given to the disorder that affects so much more than a woman's ovaries.

Later that day, a conference attendee, Lesa Childers, told me about Dr. Ronald Feinberg and his new term, *Syndrome O*. I thought, "Now, that's a good name. It sounds like something I can live with." In subsequent conversations, it became clear that Dr. Feinberg looked at this disorder from the perspective of the whole woman. We need this approach as we begin down the path of healing.

This path demands active involvement in my personal health care, and my contact with women around the world taught me that I wasn't going to have to face this battle alone. Tens of thousands of women were looking for the same answers I was, and we would look for them alongside caring physicians like Dr. Feinberg.

While many a woman has prayed for a cure for PCOS, perhaps just as many have prayed for a physician who cares—cares to stay abreast of the latest research, cares to look beyond the patient to understand the person, and cares to listen to how PCOS is affecting her life. In Dr. Feinberg, I, Lesa Childers, and countless others have found such a physician.

My challenge to you, the reader, is to open your mind to the concepts in the following pages. While it's true that Syndrome O is a disorder of the body, it is your mind that has to take the first step toward healing. It's easy to believe that Syndrome O means a lifetime of poor health, but consider this: it's just as easy to believe that you can be a Syndrome O success story.

What does a Syndrome O success story mean to you? Conceiving a child of your own? Healthy weight loss? Whatever it is, please believe that you've got a lot of people on your side, rooting for you and your good health.

We believe in you, and you should, too.

Kat Carney
Founder, SoulCysters.com
Health Anchor, CNN Headline News

HEALING
SYNDROME O

THERE'S SOMETHING ABOUT SALLY

Sally let many agonizing months go by before mustering the determination to visit my office. Once she was seated across from my desk, just a few moments passed before her eyes slowly welled with tears. "I'm so sorry for being upset, Dr. Feinberg, but this is very hard for me," she whispered. "I've come here to find out if you can help me. After going to the same doctor for twelve years, I really haven't been getting any answers. Now I feel that my body, and my life, are totally out of control."

Although not wanting to make Sally feel self-conscious, I couldn't help noticing an obvious physical characteristic—Sally's weight was well above average.

Between sobs and the wiping of tears, I listened quietly to Sally as she gradually told me more about her concerns. Sally has been happily married for eight years, and has been proud of her motherhood responsibilities for a lovable and challenging six-year-old adopted daughter. For a long time, Sally and her husband shared an intense desire to conceive a child together. They had tried for many years, but had almost given up hope. Sally expressed apprehension about how her body would respond to fertility treatments, and the couple had assumed that fertility care was beyond their financial reach.

Thankfully, Sally made an important decision to seek help and reliable information. "It took a lot of courage for me to finally come to your office," she said. "I'm not very fond of doctors. And I've been really afraid about what you might tell me." As we continued to talk, her tears dried up and she began to smile. A level of trust emerged, and she readily agreed to answer many important questions, both medical and personal in nature.

Sally told me that her last menstrual period occurred eight months ago. She couldn't remember the period prior to that. "My last doctor told me that I probably wasn't ovulating, but she really wasn't sure why. Every time I went for a visit, she ordered new blood tests. I assumed the test results were normal, since I was never told otherwise. Even though I kept gaining weight, she considered me healthy and never explained what was happening to my body. When I asked about trying to get pregnant, my doctor told me I might have to travel an hour to the large medical center for injections of fertility medicines."

After more careful questioning, I learned that many of Sally's medical problems dated back to childhood and adolescence. "I was always overweight, even as a child," she said. "As a teenager, my menstrual cycles were never regular. In high school I was actually happy to go many months between periods. Occasionally, though, I had very heavy and painful periods. No one ever told me that was bad.

"After college, I really put on a lot of weight. I tried every diet along the way, but none really worked for me." During consultation, I always ask my patients about the foods they choose to eat. Sally told me her breakfast that morning was a bagel, and that her dinner the night before consisted of a hot dog and french fries.

Describing herself as a hardworking woman, Sally told me that she balances—with some difficulty—a full-time job with a busy home life. She works for the county court, spending most of her time behind a desk, working on the computer and using the telephone. Sally enjoys her work, as well as the social interaction that her job provides. However, she wonders if her juggling act with work and home life could be interfering with her health. "I know I need to take a lot better care of myself. I need to eat better and get some exercise. But I don't have the time, and I really don't know where to begin."

In addition to her frustration with infertility and weight, Sally admitted to me a very private aspect of her diminished self-esteem—facial hair. Over the years, she has contended with increasing amounts of unwanted hair on her chin, upper lip, and on the sides of her face. "I need to shave my face almost every day. Sometimes I get very depressed about it—if my husband ever found out, I'd be so embarrassed. Recently, I've tried some laser treatments, and I think they've helped. But they're pretty expensive." I also noticed that Sally's well-groomed head of hair was thinning, perhaps more than should be expected for a thirty-year-old woman.

Sally desperately needed help strategizing her quest for improved health and fertility. Like Sally, millions of other women around the world are also struggling with similar heartbreaking problems—infertility, abnormal menstrual cycles, obesity, and nightmarish cosmetic challenges. Most of these women suffer silently, since they don't know where to turn for help. For Sally, my commitment to her as a physician is to provide education, reassurance, and an honest discussion of care options, including evaluation and treatment. In this visit and in future visits, Sally and I will set realistic goals for evaluating and improving her health. And we will work hard together to help her achieve what she and her husband most desire—a healthy pregnancy and child.

Sally came to my office searching for answers, as well as for hope. For many years she had placed her trust with a physician who didn't fully understand her problems, and who made Sally fearful about her prospects for becoming pregnant. Sally has a problem—which I call *Syndrome O*—that affects millions of women in this country and around the world. While many experts believe her problem is caused by a bad set of genes or some metabolic impairment, I prefer to describe and approach Syndrome O in a much more positive way. Just like generations of women in her family who came before her, it is very likely that she was born and blessed with a normal body and a normal reproductive system, as well as the ability to conceive and bear children.

As with many other women, Syndrome O probably began during Sally's childhood or teenage years. It was sparked by insulin and a related group of hormones that sent inappropriate signals to many parts of her body, especially organs responsible for regular menstrual cycles and reproduction. Day-to-day factors, such as less-than-optimal nutrition, reduced activity, and increased stress, fueled a vicious cycle of insulin overproduction that gradually accelerated in Sally's body. As time went on, the impact of insulin overproduction worsened her metabolism, increased her weight, and blocked her fertility. Unbeknownst to Sally, these were truly interrelated problems.

The insulin hormone family is vital to every organ of the body, yet excess amounts of these hormones have caused Sally's ovaries to become confused. In turn, her ovaries have had trouble nurturing and releasing an egg each month, an important process called *ovulation*. Without ovulation, many months can go by without a menstrual period, resulting in the inability to conceive. Tissue lining the inside of the uterus may overgrow or respond abnormally to a lack of ovulation. Sally's confused ovaries also have contributed to other difficult symptoms shared by many women with Syndrome O, such as worsening facial hair and thinning scalp hair.

Fortunately, I am convinced that women like Sally house many healthy eggs in their ovaries and that by implementing a personal action plan, Syndrome O can be healed. The challenge that lies ahead for Sally and other women with Syndrome O is to understand the unique features of how their bodies work and to create a set of strategies for breaking the cycle of insulin overproduction. This may be vitally important to you right now, in order for you to ovulate, conceive, and carry a healthy pregnancy to term. Even if getting pregnant is not your immediate goal, the Syndrome O Survival (SOS) Strategies described in chapter 9 will guide you toward fertility restoration, healthfulness, and a much better quality of life.

You may recognize Sally's plight as similar to your own. Every day, millions of women struggle with heartbreaking problems—infertility, miscarriage, obesity, and cosmetic problems that threaten their self-esteem. If that's not enough, there are the gynecologic "lady's problems"—missed menstrual cycles, heavy and unpredictable vaginal bleeding, bad reactions to birth control pills, and even unnecessary surgery. Amazingly, all of these diverse health problems are often closely related, but many doctors are not aware of the connection.

Many women who live with these personal torments suffer in silence. They might be embarrassed about the way their bodies have betrayed them with excessive weight or unsightly hair growth. They might feel that they have failed to live up to the expectations every woman has, to be able to conceive and give birth. Those who want help often don't know where to turn. For all of these women, I am here to say that there is no need to suffer alone, or in silence.

As a medical doctor, fertility specialist, and endocrinologist for more than twenty years, I have identified that women who suffer from many of these symptoms are in fact experiencing Syndrome O. *Healing Syndrome O* explains the underlying causes of these female problems, and presents options for overcoming them.

True empowerment comes through education and knowledge, and I am committed to teaching women how their metabolic and reproductive systems are intertwined. If you think about it, none of us—not you, me, or Sally—would have made it here without fertile ancestors. Women with Syndrome O need to learn that the inner workings of their metabolic and reproductive organs were inherited from a long lineage of fertile women and men. Now, their good heredity is clashing directly with modern challenges in their environment and daily lives. As my patients have acquired new information and strategies that target this concept, I've witnessed many positive transformations in health, outlook, and self-esteem. Furthermore, this healing combination of knowledge and empowerment will enhance the fertile reproductive organs that you and women like Sally were born with.

Based on what Sally has told me, many doctors would surmise that she probably has the classic clinical features of polycystic ovary disease or syndrome—a disorder "simply" described in textbooks as *hyper-*

androgenic anovulation. It is difficult for many doctors—not to mention the estimated 5 to 10 million women in the United States who suffer from different aspects of this disorder—to grasp the hormonal and reproductive concepts associated with hyperandrogenic anovulation.

Although it encompasses broader health issues for women, understanding Syndrome O means understanding many important facts about polycystic ovaries. After years of caring for women with polycystic ovaries, I've become convinced that doctors (including fertility specialists like myself) need a better way to help their patients. By writing *Healing Syndrome O,* it has not been my intent to diminish or undermine the tremendous wealth of knowledge accumulated in our textbooks and journals about polycystic ovary syndrome. But experts argue that polycystic ovary syndrome is a poorly defined clinical diagnosis and that the name is a throwback to an era when doctors believed that women's ovaries were abnormal, or even diseased.

Although thousands of women have successfully educated themselves about polycystic ovary syndrome, countless others are having trouble grasping the whys and hows of anovulation (an absence or disruption in ovulation) and hyperandrogenism (elevated "male" hormones). Furthermore, these female problems are now believed to be the consequence of a much bigger health issue affecting women *and* men throughout the world—*insulin overproduction.* Keep an open mind, and perhaps you will find that my thoughts about Syndrome O provide some new perspectives for you about the wondrous hormonal connections linking metabolism to fertility.

At the conclusion of Sally's initial visit, I reviewed with her some very important concepts about her hormones, her metabolism, and her organs of reproduction. Since Sally deserves a fighting chance to regain her fertility and her well-being, I offered her important objectives and opportunities, which will be discussed in detail in the chapters ahead. For women like Sally who have struggled for years searching for answers and who yearn for the ability to bear a healthy child, a few more honest words of wisdom lie ahead.

ONE

COULD I HAVE SYNDROME O? THE FIRST STEPS

O is the letter of the alphabet that symbolizes the cycles of life, love, and fertility. In all of the female members of the animal kingdom, the seed of life is a special O-shaped egg cell called the *oocyte* (pronounced *oh-eh-site*). Millions of microscopic oocytes live deep within an oval-shaped female organ—the ovary. As young girls approach biological adulthood, typically between the ages of ten and sixteen, both ovaries become active in maturing the oocytes and causing ovulation.

Without ovulation—the release of a mature egg from the ovary once a month—reproduction cannot easily occur. Most of the time we take the ovulation process for granted. Unfortunately, for millions of women in the United States and around the world, ovulation does not occur on a regular basis—a problem called *anovulation*. Most of these women suffer from Syndrome O, a whole body problem instigated by insulin overproduction and hormonal turmoil throughout their metabolic and reproductive systems.

So What Is Syndrome O?

Syndrome O is a reproductive problem that is unique to women of our time. Syndrome O is the World War III of hormones—causing the metabolism to be entirely out of whack, wreaking havoc with the possibility of getting and staying pregnant, and unraveling the normal sequence of hormone changes during the menstrual cycle. Syndrome O leads to disturbances within the intricate internet of hormones and glands linking metabolism and reproduction. In short, the saying "you are what you eat" holds more true today than ever before. The types and quantities of foods you choose to eat may literally be preventing you from becoming the woman you could be. This relationship between consumption and conception is the critical link that defines Syndrome O. Yet as you will read, life choices and vital factors other than food are equally important in explaining how Syndrome O develops, and how it can be healed. The basic hallmarks of Syndrome O are best defined as overnourishment (a chronic mismatch in how calories are taken in and burned, leading to insulin overproduction and a tendency toward obesity), ovarian confusion (causing the wrong balance of male and female hormones), and ovulation disruption (blocking the development and release of eggs). The basics of Syndrome O are elaborated in more detail below.

Overnourishment

There is a lot of discussion these days about fat, particularly triglycerides and cholesterol. With fat causing 50 to 60 percent of Americans to be labeled as overweight or obese—defined as the state of increased body weight caused by excessive accumulation of fat—the weight-loss industry has become a national obsession. Some view it as an embarrassing epidemic. But surprisingly, even thin people can have very abnormal fat levels circulating in their bodies. The insulin family of hormones has a major impact on fat metabolism, both in men and women. And the close connection between obesity and insulin overproduction is a proven scientific fact. As you will learn, many factors can lead to obesity, and many of the same hormone signals that lead to obesity can confuse the ovaries and prevent ovulation. Among women with Syndrome O, 80 to 90 percent are overweight or obese. For those who are thin, there is still strong evidence that excess insulin causes ovarian confusion and ovulation disruption. If ignored, many thin women with Syndrome O can gain pounds easily and eventually join the ranks of the overweight.

In reality, I prefer the word *overnourished* to the clinical term *obese*, since both thin and not-so-thin women can often be overnourished. I believe that overnourishment better describes the metabolic state of women with Syndrome O, in which the wrong quantity and quality of calories are frequently being consumed. Overnourishment also implies that the body is not sufficiently active and that the muscles are not properly burning calories. Most women who are overnourished are also overweight, but even thin women can be overnourished and suffer from Syndrome O. Overnourishment causes the ovaries to be overwhelmed with inappropriate levels of specific hormones—the insulin family of hormones—and is a major contributing factor to the other problems of ovarian confusion and ovulation disruption. Overnourishment and insulin overproduction can also lead to other Syndrome O–related health problems. In the pages ahead, there will be much discussion about the impact of overnourishment on women's ovaries, fertility, pregnancy, and health.

Ovarian Confusion

The ovaries are supposed to produce uniquely female hormones—estrogen and progesterone—in a pattern as predictable as the phases of the moon. When bombarded with inappropriate levels of insulin hormones, the ovaries become confused, producing some estrogen but very little progesterone. To make matters worse, there is a strong tendency for confused ovaries to produce slightly higher amounts of male hormones, called androgens. Androgens, like testosterone, cause all sorts of problems throughout women's bodies, particularly in the skin, leading to unsightly hair growth, acne, dark spots, and abnormal growths.

Ovulation Disruption

Deep within the ovaries are the "pearls" of mankind—tiny little eggs that lie dormant for years, waiting for the right time to emerge. The eggs live in small cystic incubators called follicles, which grow each month in response to proper hormone signals. As Syndrome O gets started, insulin signals are exaggerated and inappropriate. The insulin family of hormones *and* androgens then conspire to block normal follicle growth and the monthly release of an egg—a process that defines ovulation. In many cases, the ovaries can become mildly enlarged and polycystic. Ovulation disruption (also known as anovulation) is a *major* women's health, lifestyle, and economic problem, leading to infertility, missed menses for months at a time, and the potential for heavy, unpredictable vaginal bleeding.

Syndrome O and Syndrome X

The Syndrome O phenomenon has a common link with Syndrome X, a problem medical experts describe as a high-insulin metabolic state leading to obesity, diabetes, hypertension, and coronary artery disease. I conceived the name Syndrome O because the Syndrome X experts have not traditionally given a lot of attention to the impact of overnourishment on women's health, fertility, and pregnancy. Dr. Gerald Reaven, a distinguished professor emeritus at Stanford University, is credited with coining the term *Syndrome X*. Since the 1960s, Dr. Reaven has published hundreds of scientific studies showing that abnormal changes in metabolism, specifically caused by *insulin overproduction*, can directly influence our health. However, virtually no mention is made of the critical metabolic connections between Syndrome X, insulin, and the female reproductive system. This book aims to remedy that.

We all know that women are fundamentally different from men, both in metabolic and reproductive function. Indeed, many of the insulin-lowering strategies recommended by the Syndrome X experts could ultimately prove helpful to women. But women deserve their own evaluation and approach to care that is different from men, particularly when fertility and healthy pregnancies are at stake.

In related fashion, women are asking questions about their health and fertility in astonishing numbers. In large part this is due to the unprecedented attention paid by the media to important health topics such as infertility, pregnancy, weight management, nutrition, and body image. What causes Syndrome O? Why does it affect so many women? How is it treated? Can I achieve a healthy pregnancy? What are the health risks during pregnancy, both to my child and to me? What will happen to me as I grow older? Is Syndrome O the same as polycystic ovary syndrome? How is Syndrome O different from Syndrome X? As part of their quest for reliable information, millions of women are now seeking medical evaluation and treatment for these interrelated problems.

ORGANIZING SALLY'S SYMPTOMS

Remember the story of Sally in the introduction? Her story is similar to that of hundreds of real people who visit my clinical practice, and her symptoms are quite representative of those of countless other women affected by Syndrome O. However, most women are not generally familiar with names like Syndrome O, Syndrome X, or even polycystic ovary syndrome when they first visit their doctors.

All medical professionals are taught to identify the patient's chief complaint as a crucial part of obtaining a detailed medical history. Although Sally shared a lot of important information with me, I believe that her number one motivating reason for visiting my office related to her fertility problems. Like Sally, I have cared for thousands of women with this important chief complaint: "I want to have a baby, and I'm having trouble getting pregnant."

Infertility is defined as the inability to conceive after trying for twelve months. Sally and her husband have been married for eight years, and tried to conceive for most of that time. Sadly, no pregnancy occurred. One crucial piece of Sally's history is likely to be the culprit—a lack of menstrual periods for months at a time. This dramatic irregularity likely indicates a disruption of ovulation commonly seen with Syndrome O. But a lack of menstrual cycles (called *amenorrhea*) could also be indicative of a different diagnosis. When faced with a patient like Sally, it is imperative for a doctor to determine the cause of amenorrhea. Women who have this problem should not ignore it.

Anovulation and amenorrhea associated with Syndrome O can also lead to episodes of irregular and heavy vaginal bleeding. This may occur because the uterine lining responds to unpredictable changes in the hormonal activity of the ovaries. However, bleeding patterns such as this can also be due to other problems within the uterus, such as fibroid tumors, uterine polyps, or even cancer. As a recommendation that can't be emphasized enough, *all women with irregular bleeding patterns should be closely evaluated by a women's health professional.*

"I've gained a lot of weight" was another important concern raised by Sally, reflecting an extremely common feature of Syndrome O. However, weight gain is a multifaceted and complex problem, potentially indicative of other related health and lifestyle issues. In a recent report released by the environmental research group Worldwatch Institute, 55 percent of the U.S. population is described as overweight, with one in four adults in the United States actually considered obese. The current medical definition of obesity is based on a ratio of height and weight called BMI (body mass index). A BMI of 30 is the cutoff point between overweight and obese—a higher BMI is classified as obese. Although not every woman with Syndrome O is overweight or obese, about 80 to 90 percent of women with Syndrome O report significant problems with weight management. There is a growing understanding and appreciation of the major connections in our bodies between metabolism and reproductive function, specifically the role of the insulin hormone family. Many of the insulin changes associated with overnourishment and excess body weight have clearly been shown to have a major impact on reproductive function.

"I've developed a lot of hair on my face and chest" is another extremely common complaint of women with Syndrome O, due to the action and activity of hormones called *androgens*. Although traditionally considered to be "male hormones," it is important to realize that all women produce significant amounts of androgens, although not nearly at the same levels found in men. Women's ovaries must produce a certain amount in order to ultimately produce estrogens, or "female hormones." In fact, androgens and estrogens are *very* related. Women with Syndrome O have certain metabolic patterns of androgen activity that are different from women who don't have Syndrome O. However, the symptom doctors call *hirsutism* (excess body hair) can be caused by significant medical problems unrelated to Syndrome O. A complaint of hirsutism, particularly if abrupt in onset or severity, requires close medical evaluation.

The Syndrome O–related problems expressed by Sally—amenorrhea, infertility, weight gain, and hirsutism—are such important topics that separate detailed chapters have been devoted to each. It is important to remember that all of these clinical problems reflect the basic hallmarks of Syndrome O—Overnourishment, Ovarian confusion, and Ovulation disruption—which are all instigated by the overproduction of insulin.

If I Think I Have Syndrome O, What Type of Doctor Should I See?

Finding the right doctor to evaluate a diverse set of symptoms is a challenging feat. Doctors with different specialties and interests, such as internists, family practitioners, obstetrician/gynecologists, dermatologists, and endocrinologists, may commonly see patients with Syndrome O. It can often be difficult for many busy physicians to understand or assess the "bigger picture" of Syndrome O.

Most people think of doctors who practice endocrinology, my chosen specialty, as "gland doctors." That is generally an accurate point of view. As new knowledge accumulated in the medical sciences over the past one hundred years, specialization in specific endocrine problems affecting men, women, and children became necessary. There are now different types of clinical endocrinologists—those within the field of adult internal medicine (*medical* endocrinologists), those in the specialty of children's medicine (*pediatric* endocrinologists), and others, like myself, in obstetrics, gynecology, and women's health (*reproductive* endocrinologists). The broad endeavor of endocrinology has also captured the attention of many talented research scientists, who diligently contribute vast amounts of new information through their studies in cell biology, molecular biology, genetics, biochemistry, physiology, and pharmacology.

Endocrinologists, both in clinical practice and research, spend a great deal of time thinking about glands and the hormone substances produced by glands. Not every woman who has Syndrome O or related symptoms needs to be under the direct care of a clinical endocrinologist. However, since it is so closely linked to glandular and hormonal function, endocrinologists are commonly asked to evaluate women with Syndrome O. Because the majority of women with Syndrome O tend to have symptoms directly related to their reproductive organs, it is very common for women to first seek help from their gynecologist, or possibly from a reproductive endocrinologist.

Reproductive endocrinologists are trained as specialists in fertility care, and they have usually devoted two to three *extra* years of clinical training and research in addition to their four-year residencies in obstetrics and gynecology. To become board-certified, reproductive endocrinologists must pass four different rigorous tests to demonstrate their scientific and clinical competence in the care of women with diverse medical problems—including infertility. Many become recertified on an annual basis. With up-to-date expertise in women's health and endocrinology, they are particularly well educated to provide consultation to women with Syndrome O.

THE INITIAL OFFICE VISIT

When I meet patients, I have many individualized questions to ask—both medical and nonmedical. While information concerning the reproductive system is certainly very important to ascertain, I also want to know some significant aspects about these women's lives—how they spend their days, the foods they like to eat, whether they participate in physical activities, their relationship with their spouses or partners, the stresses they have at work or home, their life goals, and their self-esteem. Activities, environment, and lifestyle choices are important factors in our quest to better understand the diverse challenges of Syndrome O.

Clinical endocrinologists tend to be very global in their evaluation, since hormonal fluctuations can influence the body in many different ways. Following a thorough initial consultation, the doctor will perform a detailed physical examination, which is mandatory for establishing a diagnosis of Syndrome O. Particular attention is given to height and weight, blood pressure and heart rate, the size of the thyroid gland (an important metabolism regulator), examination of the heart, lungs, breasts, and abdomen, and a survey of the skin. For women with menstrual cycle irregularity or fertility issues, a pelvic examination and ultrasound is often highly informative. The ultrasound is usually performed transvaginally and most women don't consider it to be an uncomfortable experience. This type of ultrasound provides excellent information about the appearance of the uterus and ovaries. Women with Syndrome O will, in 70 to 80 percent of cases, have ovaries that contain many tiny follicle *cysts*. Although this is a common ovarian appearance, it is not required for the diagnosis of Syndrome O. For patients in my practice, transvaginal ultrasound also serves as an outstanding way to teach women more about their reproductive organs.

You may already have come to realize that Syndrome O is not a simple problem, nor are there simple answers for healing many of the different aspects of Syndrome O that likely affect you. This box lists twenty-five important personal questions for you to consider and tries to organize them within the Syndrome O hallmarks of overnourishment, ovarian confusion, and ovulation disruption. In the chapters ahead, it should become clearer to you why these questions are relevant. As you read more, refer back to these questions frequently and feel free to use them as a guide before and during your visits with doctors and other health professionals.

COULD I HAVE SYNDROME O?

QUESTIONS TO ASK MYSELF WHEN I VISIT THE DOCTOR

Questions related to overnourishment and insulin overproduction:

1. Do I know my body mass index (BMI)?
2. Is my BMI in the overweight or obese range?
3. Do I frequently miss meals, especially breakfast?
4. Do I tend to eat too much at other meals, especially late in the day?
5. Do I frequently crave sweets, breads, pasta, rice, or potatoes?
6. Have I gained weight, especially around my abdomen and waist, over the past year? Five years? Ten years?
7. Do I gain weight back after dieting, and then some extra (the yo-yo effect)?
8. Do I have many skin tags and/or dark patches on my skin?
9. Do I have a family history of obesity, diabetes, or cardio-vascular disease?
10. Has a doctor ever told me that my fat, cholesterol, sugar, or insulin levels are abnormal? Or that I have "a little" diabetes, spikes of low blood sugar (*hypoglycemia*), or high blood pressure?

Questions related to ovarian confusion:

11. Do I have worsening hair growth on my face and/or body?
12. Is my scalp hair thinning or balding?
13. Do I have acne and/or oily skin?
14. Were my menstrual periods irregular as a teenager? Did I go through puberty earlier than most other girls my age?
15. Has a doctor ever told me that my androgen (male hormone) levels are abnormal?

Questions related to ovulation disruption:

16. Are my menstrual periods routinely more than thirty-five days apart? Or shorter than twenty-one days?
17. Do I get unpredictable episodes of heavy, prolonged bleeding?
18. Have I been trying to get pregnant for over a year without success?
19. Have I had any miscarriages recently, or in the past?
20. Has a doctor prescribed fertility medicines to me without success?

General approach-to-life questions:

21. Do I view my life, career, family, and relationships as a burden or an opportunity?
22. Am I frequently sad or depressed?
23. Do I wish I had more time and energy to improve my health and well being?
24. Do I believe that there are people out there who can help me?
25. Do I believe that I can help myself by helping others?

Blood tests are usually another important part of any endocrinologic evaluation. Any hormone that has proven to have clinical significance can be measured in a laboratory. Doctors who practice endocrinology rely heavily on the measurements of certain hormones that circulate throughout the bloodstream. Sometimes it is important to measure specific hormones during a certain time of day, such as first thing in the morning before a meal (i.e., a *fasting* blood level). When evaluating women for Syndrome O, it is often helpful to measure blood levels of hormones related to metabolism and reproductive function. While these blood tests do not necessarily confirm or refute a diagnosis of Syndrome O, they can help endocrinologists fine-tune their clinical impression after consultation, examination, and ultrasound. In addition, clinical blood tests can help doctors tell if you're at risk for other related health issues, such as diabetes and heart disease.

Many women with Syndrome O are willing to accept the fact that their "bad" genes determine their fate. I have a very different philosophy. I strongly believe that women with Syndrome O actually have an excellent set of genes. Unfortunately, in a society blessed with modern conveniences and the seemingly unending availability of food and sedentary activity, the wonderful intricate pattern of genes and hormone signals linking metabolism and reproduction in women will often go awry. With more and more people suffering from obesity, diabetes, and heart disease, it is possible that in ten years, Syndrome O will affect 20 to 25 percent of the U.S. female population. Heredity versus environment? Determinism versus free will? Passiveness versus proactive change? Only Sally and women like her can decide for themselves what their personal philosophy will be to overcome the Syndrome O risks to their fertility and health.

You may be experiencing many of the problems that Sally and other women with Syndrome O face. You probably feel overwhelmed and saddened, but may not know how to get started on the path toward wellness. Hopefully, this book contains some of the answers you are looking for.

As you read through *Healing Syndrome O*, keep an eye out for different Syndrome O issues that could be important to you. No woman has the exact same set of symptoms, yet countless women share the desire to achieve a healthy pregnancy. Although this book is especially committed to overcoming fertility and pregnancy problems for women with Syndrome O, I hope it will also help the multitude of women who are considering getting pregnant in the future.

Likewise, women who are beyond childbearing years may find solace in understanding the source of problems they might have experienced in the past. They may also be able to offer newfound wisdom about Syndrome O to loved ones who currently desire children. Most important, my goal is to lift your body and spirit toward many years of healthy and happy living.

KEY MOTIVATIONAL POINTS

- Syndrome O affects millions of women like Sally in the United States and around the world. It represents a clash of good heredity and fertility with modern challenges, such as quality and quantity of food choices, limited physical activity, and extra stress. Syndrome O is not a consequence of "bad" genes, but of a changing environment that all people must adapt to.

- Syndrome O is unique to women and is best defined as a triad of overnourishment, ovarian confusion, and ovulation disruption. These three basic components, caused by insulin overproduction, contribute to common Syndrome O problems: infertility, miscarriage, weight gain, excess hair growth, irregular or absent menstrual cycles, and many cases of abnormal vaginal bleeding.

- Syndrome O includes the high insulin health consequences of Syndrome X that affect millions of women and men: cardiovascular disease, insulin resistance and diabetes, hypertension, and obesity. Unfortunately, many teens, twenty- and thirty-something women are already afflicted with these metabolic problems, which are typically associated with older individuals.

- If you think you have Syndrome O, use this book as a guide to help you prioritize your Syndrome O concerns and approach to care. Then seek out a trusted physician who can take a thorough history and evaluate you properly. Based on your chief complaint, there are many different specialists and subspecialists who can provide you with state-of-the-art treatment options, such as fertility care.
- Keep an open mind and a positive outlook. There are dedicated professionals out there who can help you, if you are committed to helping yourself.

TWO

HORMONES, INSULIN, AND FERTILITY: WHAT'S HAPPENING IN YOUR BODY

YOU STARTED LIFE FROM A GOOD EGG!

Your life has been in the making for more years than you think. When your mother was a tiny fetus in her mother's womb, swarms of undeveloped precursor eggs called germ cells (*germ* meaning germinate) congregated in two specific spots in her fetal abdomen, giving rise to her ovaries. The particular egg destined to become *you,* along with millions of others, were then protected and nourished by special ovary cells. By the time your mother was born, many of her original egg cells had withered away—a normal and important egg selection process that continues through adulthood. Fortunately, tens of thousands of other eggs continued to live within her ovaries—including the healthy one from which you came to be.

Within a protective ovarian incubator called the *follicle,* your egg remained dormant for many years. Like thousands of other sister eggs housed in separate follicles, your egg was initially a clone of your mother's genes. It contained DNA and chromosome pairs identical to all of the other cells throughout her body. Gradually, as your mother grew from childhood into adolescence, she experienced major whole-body changes, initiated primarily by surges of hormones from her brain. For the minute eggs and follicles within your mother's ovaries, a seismic hormonal earthquake was about to commence.

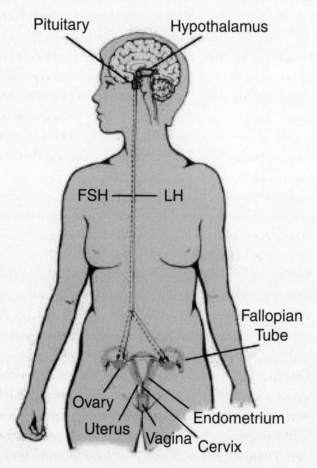

Puberty starts when unique hormones from the brain's hypothalamus are released as potent informational bursts, with just the right timing and intensity. The pituitary gland, a pea-sized master gland located behind the nose, promptly receives and responds to those signals by directing many functions throughout the body, including physical growth and maturation. Two specific pituitary hormones—follicle stimulating hormone (FSH) and luteinizing hormone (LH)—pulsate into the bloodstream according to the brain's instructions. During a woman's entire reproductive life both FSH and LH carry instructions to the ovaries, directing orderly follicle growth, egg development, ovulation, and preparation for pregnancy.

Puberty-related hormones in girls and boys are designed to stimulate growth and development of the entire body, leading to the capability for reproduction. Scientists have spent years trying to learn about the circuitry in the brain responsible for starting puberty and regulating menstrual cycles. We don't have all the answers, but nutrition, fitness, and general health are vital factors. The connections of brain and body to the menstrual cycle are particularly relevant to Syndrome O. Curiously, women with Syndrome O always experienced puberty (sometimes even on the early side), yet typically did not menstruate regularly, as adolescents. This is a common but often overlooked early sign of confused ovaries and ovulation disruption in teenage girls. The pituitary hormones FSH and LH were trying to do their job of stimulating ovarian follicles in a cyclical fashion, but the insulin hormone family was getting in the way.

As your mother's adolescence progressed, not only did she grow taller and develop breasts, it is likely that she experienced initial menstrual bleeding between the ages of ten and sixteen. Breast growth and menstrual bleeding are related events, since they predictably occur once the ovaries produce *estrogen*. Specialized *granulosa cells* within maturing ovarian follicles produce remarkable quantities of estrogen. Granulosa cells are also responsible for nourishing the egg and stimulating egg development when proper signals from the brain, pituitary gland, and other glands are put into motion.

It is not likely that you were conceived from the very first mature egg released during your mother's first cycle of ovulation. Based on our knowledge of ovarian physiology, your specific egg and follicle began awakening from their dormant state about one year before you were born. Despite years of research and speculation, no one is exactly sure what combinations of signals are necessary to initiate this wakeup call. Along with your egg and follicle, a few others also started to develop, replaying a fascinating competition for follicle dominance that occurred on a monthly schedule.

Unless you have a fraternal twin, your egg and follicle clearly won the monthly contest for egg release (i.e., ovulation) from your mother's ovaries. Your follicle, along with the granulosa cells inside, responded best to your mother's FSH during the month you were conceived. Other follicles in the group fell behind in the growth contest and slowly withered away. Inside of your follicle, granulosa cells were busy producing enzymes to help your egg exit through its follicle wall. A major midcycle surge in the bloodstream from another vital pituitary hormone, LH, induced your egg to undergo a maturing process and further prepared your follicle for ovulation.

The environment in your winning follicle encouraged your egg to undergo a major transformation. As ovulation approached, your egg truly germinated by beginning a genetic event called *meiosis.* No other cell in the female body is capable of meiosis. As meiosis progressed, your egg matured and efficiently eliminated one complete set of your mother's chromosomes. Meiosis was the foremost event necessary for you to become a unique human being. For successful conception, which was destined to happen just hours later, your egg needed to make room for a new set of chromosomes arriving from your father.

Ovulation allowed your egg, along with some attached granulosa cells, to exit the follicle incubator at the proper time. Just after ovulation, but before fertilization, the delicate fingers of your mother's fallopian tube embraced your egg and gently pulled it into the passageway leading to the uterus. Once inside this canal, the egg was nourished by special fallopian tube fluids, allowing normal fertilization and growth. The sperm that fertilized your egg also had a long developmental journey, ending in the fallopian tube where it joined your egg. Since that single sperm provided you with a crucial second set of genes and chromosomes (it also underwent meiosis in your father's testes), both sperm and egg were equal winners in determining your genetic destiny.

During the first few days following conception, your free-floating egg (now called a *zygote*) provided much of its own metabolic energy, allowing it to rapidly divide as it moved down the fallopian tube. One egg cell soon became two cells, then four, then eight, and within five days after conception, you became an embryonic ball of cells in your mother's uterus, preparing for attachment. The lining of your mother's

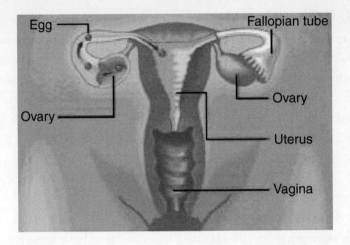

The female reproductive system. On a monthly schedule, a mature egg will develop and be released from one ovary following ovulation. During a cycle of conception, the egg will undergo fertilization within the fallopian tube. The fertilized egg (zygote) then undergoes rapid cell division. Once fertilized, the early embryo migrates into the uterus, where implantation and pregnancy development occur.

uterus, the *endometrium,* was hormonally primed by estrogen, and then stimulated with *progesterone,* a second vital ovarian hormone. Progesterone is produced in large quantities by the granulosa cells remaining in the follicle after ovulation.

Preparation of the uterine lining for your mother's pregnancy involved a series of synchronized steps in advance of your embryo's *implantation.* Physicians and scientists are profoundly interested in gaining more knowledge about implantation, since this vital process greatly affects the success of low- and high-tech fertility treatments and the maintenance of a healthy pregnancy. An important research mission in the world of reproductive medicine is to avoid pregnancy complications related to implantation abnormalities, such as miscarriage, pregnancy-induced hypertension (toxemia), fetal growth retardation, and stillbirth.

Within a few weeks after implantation, your own fetal form began to take shape. Sensitive ultrasound can now verify fetal heart activity approximately four weeks after conception. Many other organs were also forming during your early fetal life, including a whole new generation of germ cells destined to provide you with the seedlings for your future children. Despite ongoing frustrations you may have had with ovarian confusion and ovulation disruption, it is 99 percent likely you were born with healthy ovaries containing thousands of normal follicles and eggs. Therefore, our mission is to help your ovaries, eggs, and follicles work properly, and to make your body fertile.

MAKING YOUR OVARIES WORK

The phenomenon of Syndrome O underscores how sensitive your fertility can be to a multitude of internal and external signals. Although the impact of Syndrome O upon fertility involves the entire body, we must give major attention to the ovaries because the development and release of healthy eggs is paramount to successful reproduction. Since you were likely born with normal ovaries, it is also likely you were born with normal genes, i.e. "the right stuff," to make your ovaries function properly. "So what has gone wrong?" you might ask. "And why aren't my ovaries working the way they are supposed to?"

Before addressing those crucial questions, let's first consider some facts about the specialized communities of cells designed to work together within your ovaries. In addition to the eggs and granulosa cells protected within thousands of tiny follicles, the ovaries contain other important hormone-producing cells within their connective tissue scaffold. These are called *theca cells* and *stromal cells*, and they are particularly sensitive to imbalances in the insulin family of hormones. Unlike the granulosa cells, which produce estrogen, theca cells and stromal cells produce *androgen* hormones, such as testosterone.

Compared to women, men have much higher levels of testosterone in their bloodstream, which is why androgens are commonly considered "male hormones." Nevertheless, all women must have androgen-producing cells in their ovaries because androgens are used by the granulosa cells to synthesize estrogen. Just one special enzyme in the granulosa cells, called *aromatase,* is required to rapidly change the chemistry of male hormones (i.e., androgens) into female hormones (i.e., estrogens). Progesterone is also a unique and vital hormone of the ovaries, produced by granulosa cells after ovulation.

Like every other organ in the body, the ovaries have a rich network of blood vessels—arteries that deliver oxygen, nutrients, and hormones, veins that send by-products and ovarian hormones exiting to the rest of the body, and lymph channels that maintain fluid balance. The flow of hormone signals in and out of the ovaries via the bloodstream allows for an efficient communication network between the ovaries and other organs of the body. For women, the ovaries are a vital part of the *glandular internet,* a delicate network of hormones allowing all organs and cells of the body to converse with one another. When hormonal cross-talk throughout the body leads to follicle growth, ovulation, and a healthy pregnancy, it is likely that the glandular internet is functioning efficiently.

Both ovaries are part of the finely tuned glandular internet because they are wired via the bloodstream to give and receive hormone signals. FSH and LH from the pituitary are paramount, since without these hormones pulsing into the bloodstream the ovaries will not function properly. Part of a woman's genetic program provides for granulosa and theca cells to be responsive to specific amounts of FSH and LH. Like all hormones, FSH and LH function by a lock-and-key mechanism, attaching to receptor proteins in ovarian cells. FSH and LH receptors are the "e-mail addresses," or specific docking stations, for FSH and LH within ovarian cells. Thousands of other unique receptor proteins are present throughout organs of the glandular internet, providing the basis for how the endocrine system functions.

Fluctuating amounts of FSH and LH in the bloodstream determine how active the ovaries will be in producing androgens, estrogens, and progesterone throughout the menstrual cycle. Just the right balance of FSH and LH are also required to induce normal follicle growth and egg development. More recent discoveries have shown that developing ovarian follicles transmit many crucial hormone signals through the bloodstream back to the brain and pituitary, thus regulating FSH and LH levels. Endocrinologists refer to this back-and-forth communication channel as the hypothalamic (brain)-pituitary-ovarian axis, or HPO circle. It is the backbone of human reproduction.

Neither the ovaries, nor the HPO circle exist in isolation. With the bloodstream constantly transporting thousands of hormones through-out the body, the HPO circle both requires and is vulnerable to other signals from the glandular internet. Have you had a stressful day? Your adrenal glands might be pouring some extra stress hormones—like cortisol, epinephrine, and even androgens—into your bloodstream. Did you forget to eat breakfast? Your HPO circle might not be happy with your low blood sugar, nor jolting peaks and valleys of insulin when you do sit down to a meal. How about that late night snack? Depending on the quality and quantity of the snack, some extra in-sulin was likely coursing through your body all night long.

Fortunately, the brain, pituitary, and ovaries are quite resilient to most of the hormonal consequences of daily living. After all, human beings have evolved over the ages to withstand more severe stressors than a bad day at work or some poorly timed meals. However, mod-ern humans in many societies, particularly in the United States, have developed chronic twenty-first-century patterns of overnourish-ment, underactivity, poor sleep, and stress. For many men and women,

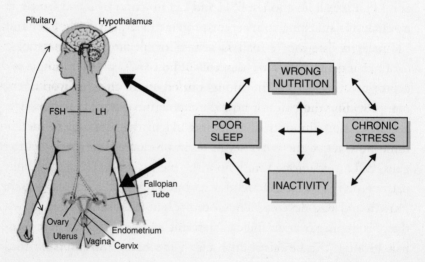

the impact of these life habits may have begun years ago, during their teenage years or even in childhood. Syndrome O is one significant consequence of the modern ongoing clash between environment and genetics. For the millions of women around the world affected by Syndrome O, their ovaries provide a valuable lesson of how bad things can happen to good organs.

The Syndrome O Threats to Your Body

Hormonal misfires within the glandular internet can upset the delicate flow of signals required for healthy follicle and egg development. For women who are trying to conceive, *ovulation disruption* becomes the most significant roadblock. Although it is well known to many women that doctors can prescribe medications to induce ovulation, these medications do not readily correct the other significant aspects of Syndrome O—*ovarian confusion* and *overnourishment*. Furthermore, should a pregnancy occur, miscarriage and other pregnancy problems occur more frequently for women with Syndrome O, unless strategic life-management changes have been instituted prior to conception.

Metabolic hormones such as insulin are profoundly important to women. Based on heredity and environment, the entire insulin family of hormones is constantly exerting an impact on the female reproductive system. Heredity created a genetic plan for your ovaries, follicles, and eggs to respond to insulin in a certain programmed fashion. The genetic plan was carried in the DNA and chromosomes of your winning egg and sperm. It is based solely on what worked successfully for your parents, grandparents, and countless generations before them. With some wiggle room, your environment and life choices must agree with that genetic plan in order to overcome Syndrome O.

It is not difficult to identify the modern environmental factors that interfere with the glandular internet and lead to worsening Syndrome O problems: sugar and fat consumption, stress, inactivity, and inadequate sleep. These factors conspire to promote overnourishment, a common state in modern society whereby more food calories are ingested than burned. Chronic overnourishment leads to a state of insulin overproduction, which in most men and women results in weight gain. Continued weight gain usually means that unused calories are being stored as fat, a useful biological insurance policy that allowed our ancestors to survive a famine. Thin and normal weight individuals can also be overnourished, and even though they do not readily form excess fat, they may well have insulin levels that exceed their genetic predispostion.

When too much food is consumed and you burn an inadequate amount of calories, overnourishment persists and insulin levels continue to increase. As a chronic problem, overnourishment often coexists with obesity and insulin resistance. Insulin, along with other insulin-related hormones, affect the HPO circle at several key steps:

1. Disrupting the delicate balance in the brain's hypothalamus, causing abnormal pulsations of FSH and LH from the pituitary gland.
2. Inducing the theca cells and stromal cells of the ovaries to produce excess androgens.
3. Mimicking the action of FSH within the follicle, leading to inappropriate and inadequate follicle growth (i.e., growth of polycysts).
4. Blocking enzymes needed to break the follicle wall at the time of ovulation.

Overproduction of insulin causes these problems to occur, although the time course may vary significantly based on how severe and how chronically the ovaries have been affected.

Experts from many different specialties of health care have concluded that insulin overproduction is both incited and exacerbated by a combination of factors, including those mentioned earlier. For women trying to break their own personal cycle of overnourishment, ovarian confusion, and ovulation disruption, here is a more detailed discussion of some common and important lifestyle factors that can wreak havoc on your fertility, reproductive system, and general health.

- *Sugar.* Every cell in the human body needs a simple sugar called glucose for survival. It is made by plants, through a miraculous process known as photosynthesis, which combines water, carbon dioxide, and light energy into sugar energy blocks called *carbohydrates.* Much of our glucose sources derive from the sugar cane plant, from which we refine a sweet-tasting substance known as *sucrose.* Enzymes in our saliva, stomach, and intestines readily convert sucrose into glucose, and the sugar is rapidly absorbed into the bloodstream. Soon after eating sugar, the pancreas responds promptly and vigorously by pouring insulin into the bloodstream. Insulin is required to shuttle glucose from the bloodstream into all cells. If many cells, such as muscle and fat cells, are insulin-resistant, insulin must be oversecreted by the pancreas in order to compensate. Type 2 diabetes results when the body's demand for insulin is overbearing and the pancreas can no longer keep up.
- *Sugar water (soft drinks and unnatural "juices").* Bottling companies have been selling billions of bottles of sugar water for many years to an unsuspecting public throughout the world. A typical twelve-ounce can of soda may contain more than 200 calories from sugar. That's equal to about fifteen teaspoons of table sugar. Many brands of regular cola, iced tea, and juices are further fortified with caffeine, a compound with known addictive qualities. Many people who claim that they don't eat very much consume several servings of sugar water each day, adding much unnecessary fuel to their overnourished bodies. It is guaranteed that insulin will surge after a jolt of sugar water.
- *Starches.* Many edible plants, such as potatoes, rice, wheat, and corn, synthesize and compact sugar into larger molecules, providing the denser forms of carbohydrate found in breads, pasta, and many other foods. Nutritionists commonly

score carbohydrates based on their *glycemic index,* which gives
a rating of the quantity of glucose being released into the
bloodstream. Starchy foods tend to have higher glycemic indices than most fruits and vegetables. The quantity and quality of starch carbohydrates that are necessary in the diet has
spurred a major debate among scientists, physicians, and dieticians. However, the debates usually fail to discuss the
unique requirements and fertility goals of women with Syndrome O. In this author's opinion, neither an ultra-high nor
ultra-low carbohydrate diet is likely to be beneficial for
women trying to outsmart Syndrome O.

- *Funny fats.* The twentieth century produced many marvels
  and inventions relevant to food preparation and safe storage.
  One innovation of questionable health value was hydrogenation, a chemical process introduced in 1911 by Procter &
  Gamble, permitting the conversion of vegetable oils into long
  chain molecules resembling animal fats. There is now widespread concern that partial hydrogenation of different vegetable
  oils (as in shortening and margarine) results in a modified fat
  molecule (*trans* fat) that wreaks havoc with human metabolism when ingested in excess. The problem lies in defining
  what constitutes excessive trans fat intake and determining
  whether some people are affected more than others. Different theories suggest that trans fats can compete with vital fat-
  metabolizing enzymes and that trans fats infiltrate the body's
  essential fatty components, such as fat cells and cell membranes. By distorting the lipid bilayer of cell membranes that
  houses insulin receptors, trans fats may impede cells' responsiveness to insulin. When cells can't react to insulin signals efficiently, both insulin resistance and insulin overproduction are
  the consequences. It is recommended that trans fat intake be
  strictly limited to less than 2 grams per day. Americans readily ingest five to ten times that amount or more on a daily basis. Unlike numerous essential vegetable and animal fats found
  in nature, there is no evidence that any specific quantity of

trans fats is required for normal body functions. Food labels will soon contain detailed information about the quantity of trans fats per serving, along with other nutrient information.

- *Screen demons.* Our genetic heritage did not anticipate the impact that "screen machines" would have on our modern tendency toward inactivity. Screen machines are everywhere now—at work, at home, in restaurants, and even in doctors' waiting rooms. Have you counted the number of hours per week that you spend watching TV, reading and answering e-mail, surfing the Internet, paying your bills online, reading articles, and perhaps playing some video games? Millions of men and women spend most of their days at work in front of a computer screen. All this sitting around means that the brain might be active, but that most of the body's muscles are not. While you stare at a screen demon, calories are being burned very slowly by the rest of your body. Reversing a sedentary life is one of the biggest challenges to women with Syndrome O.

- *Stressful sitting.* When not staring at a screen machine, we spend countless other hours sitting in cars and in other modes of transportation. In many instances, the sitting is not so pleasant, creating additional stress in our lives. For myself, I created a lot of personal stress during my hours of interaction with my Apple PowerBook screen demon, knowing I was months behind in my writing endeavors. The impact of inactivity, and the inherent additional stress it creates, leads to muscle underuse, excessive cortisol secretion from the adrenal glands, and a worsening of insulin resistance. There are no easy answers to these apparent stressful necessities of life in the twenty-first century.

- *Fitful sleeping.* Inadequate hours of sleep, along with suboptimal sleep quality, lead to further stress-related augmentation of insulin resistance. The incidence of a serious sleep disorder, known as *sleep apnea,* has been identified in many insulin-resistant individuals, including women with Syndrome O.

Controlled weight loss, changes in dietary habits, and exercise
have all been shown to improve sleep quality. A reduction in
other stressful activities and interactions, whether at home or
work, will also fortify sleep habits. Perhaps you are "sweating
the small stuff," as author Richard Carlson would argue, resulting in unnecessary angst before bedtime. Never underestimate
the value of a good night's sleep and the impact that will have
on your reproductive organs.

ANDROGENS AND OVARIAN CONFUSION

Androgens such as testosterone are fundamental hormones for successful reproduction in men *and* women, and androgens are constantly being produced within all women's ovaries. Under normal
circumstances, pulsing messages of LH and FSH from the pituitary
gland, along with the insulin family of hormones, modulate the
quantity of androgens that are produced by ovarian theca and stromal
cells (these cells defined previously on page 26). In women with Syndrome O, androgen production is accentuated due to insulin overproduction. This interaction is the hallmark of ovarian confusion.

Deep inside the ovarian theca and stromal cells are small enzyme
factories that spend twenty-four hours a day converting cholesterol
from the bloodstream into androgens. Ironically, it is the so-called
"bad" LDL-cholesterol that is required for those key enzyme steps.
Androgen-producing enzymes are also particularly sensitive to LH
and insulin. Women share with men the exact enzymes to produce
androgens from LDL-cholesterol but in a sense, women's ovarian enzymes have evolved beyond those of men.

When the right balance of androgens, insulin, FSH, and LH flow
into the tiny ovarian follicles, the granulosa cells surrounding the egg
are called to action. The unique enzyme aromatase (which the male
testis doesn't have) becomes activated and estrogens are readily produced from androgens. The main active estrogen made is *estradiol,* and
it can be measured. Fertility doctors test estradiol blood levels fre-

quently for their patients when ovulation induction treatments are under way and follicles start to grow (discussed in chapters 4 and 5).

For all women, heredity determines the activity of androgen-producing enzymes and the ability of the granulosa cells to produce estrogen. And it is an absolute truth that androgens are vital to all female reproductive functions. Along with that, tiny ovarian follicles have a certain zone of sensitivity and dependence upon specific amounts of androgens, insulin, FSH, and LH. With the proper balance of these hormones, granulosa cells will grow and produce estrogen properly. Follicles will grow in a consistent and cyclical pattern when the right hormone signals are received.

All reproductive-age women, whether affected by Syndrome O or not, have predictably maintained thousands of healthy dormant follicles since birth. Most of these are microscopic and can't be seen by

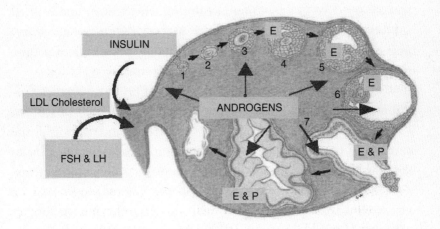

Cross-section schematic drawing of a human ovary, demonstrating the flow of insulin, FSH, and LH hormones into the ovary from the bloodstream. These hormones, along with LDL cholesterol, stimulate enzymes to produce androgens within ovarian theca and stromal cells. Androgens are then used by the granulosa cells in the developing follicles (numbered 1 through 6) to produce increasing amounts of estrogen (E). After ovulation (#7), the follicle becomes a corpus luteum, synthesizing progesterone (P). Androgens are also required for this process. If excess androgens are produced, ovarian confusion and ovulation disruption will result. Androgens will also leave the ovaries via the bloodstream to have effects elsewhere in the body. Picture of ovary courtesy of www.cells.hihome.com

ultrasound. Women with Syndrome O have inherited a genetic makeup rendering their follicles and ovaries exquisitely sensitive to the essential hormones of reproduction—insulin, androgens, FSH, and LH. This pattern of heredity is not unique to one ethnic group or culture. It is present in many millions of women around the world and from virtually all ethnic backgrounds. What might then explain this worldwide "epidemic" of Syndrome O?

We know that throughout the evolution and history of womankind, food was much less plentiful and food choices were limited in quantity and quality. Activity levels were much greater. As a result, insulin levels were much lower, particularly when compared to many parts of the world today. Yet our species survived, as women and men passed their strong insulin-sensitive genes to subsequent generations. We all started life from a good egg, as did our ancestors.

The most fertile women through the ages were those who had a high abundance of ovarian follicles, as well as ovaries that were particularly sensitive to a low insulin environment. These same women had follicles that functioned best with just the right amounts of androgens, FSH, and LH. Syndrome O is certainly not a freak of nature, but more a phenomenon of good heredity going awry.

With this information, the Syndrome O hallmark of ovarian confusion becomes much easier to comprehend. For millions of women with Syndrome O throughout the United States and the world, the amounts of insulin and androgens flowing into their ovarian follicles likely exceeds their inherited genetic program. As a result, key enzyme systems within the theca, stromal, and granulosa cells become overwhelmed and poisoned. This halts follicle and egg development and contributes to an accelerated death process in otherwise healthy follicles called *atresia*.

After months or years of insulin overproduction, numerous small and partially developed atretic follicles will accumulate. In many women with Syndrome O, this can cause the ovaries to become slightly enlarged, taking on a polycystic appearance on ultrasound. Thus the term polycystic ovaries. For many years, doctors believed that the ovaries were primarily diseased in such women. Medical textbooks today still refer to polycystic ovary disease, or syndrome, and sometimes to the name Stein-Leventhal.

In the 1930s, two Chicago gynecologists—Drs. Stein and Leventhal—first described seven cases of polycystic ovaries. They performed abdominal surgery on those women, believing that ovarian tumors might be present (there was no ultrasound in that era). The doctors were intrigued to learn that the portions of ovaries they removed contained multiple, partially developed small follicles, but certainly no cancer. The clear connection between polycystic ovaries and insulin overproduction remained undiscovered for about sixty years after these original Stein and Leventhal observations.

In more chronic and severe cases of Syndrome O, the poisoned and atretic follicles become replaced within the ovaries by connective tissue stromal cells. These additional stromal cells produce androgens and are sensitive to insulin, thus fueling a worsening vicious cycle. In this setting, the ovaries may lose their polycystic appearance, whether by ultrasound imaging or under the microscope. Thus, it is folly to assume that Syndrome O requires the presence of polycystic ovaries.

Is ovarian confusion reversible? To the extent that it results primarily from insulin overproduction, the answer is yes. The extent of reversibility may depend on how long the ovaries have been bombarded with excess insulin and androgens. Some doctors argue strenuously for the aggressive use of medications, while others like myself prefer life-management strategies as first-line approaches. Reversing ovarian confusion takes time, however, and some drug treatments are incompatible with attempting pregnancy. Others may enhance the likelihood of conceiving if they are monitored properly.

Androgens can have far-reaching effects throughout a woman's body, leading to some dreaded cosmetic nightmares—unwanted hair growth on the face, chest, and abdomen, thinning hair on the scalp, acne, and oily skin. Chapter 10 will be devoted to a detailed discussion of these problems. Although the ovaries have typically been blamed for contributing to excess androgens throughout the body, it is really insulin overproduction that underlies this issue.

Insulin excess is the major culprit causing both ovarian and adre-

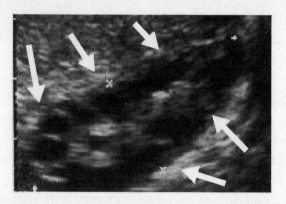

Ultrasound image of a "polycystic" appearing ovary. Arrows point to multiple tiny cyst-like follicles noted throughout the periphery of the ovary. These tiny follicles have usually developed in response to an overabundant amount of insulin and androgens. Many women with Syndrome O do not have classic "polycystic" appearing ovaries, although the triad of Overnourishment, Ovarian Confusion, and Ovulation Disruption are present.

nal gland androgens to be overproduced. At the same time, chronic insulin overload instructs the liver to dramatically reduce its synthesis of *sex hormone binding globulin* (SHBG). This vital sponge protein binds and carries androgens and estrogens throughout the bloodstream, carefully controlling how much is released to different organs. A low amount of SHBG means that higher amounts of "free," or unbound, androgen in the bloodstream can attack the skin, scalp, hair follicles, and even the ovaries themselves. Low SHBG and high "free" androgen blood levels are found in most women with Syndrome O. Furthermore, a low SHBG level in men and women has been widely recognized as a marker for insulin resistance and overproduction.

Medications that help sensitize the body to insulin can achieve dramatic short-term reductions in insulin and "free" androgen levels. Concomitantly, normal follicle growth and ovulation can occur when these medicines are taken, suggesting that ovarian confusion and ovulation disruption have been temporarily improved. Insulin sensitizers allow the body to utilize insulin more efficiently and are most commonly prescribed to people with type 2, or adult-onset, diabetes. In recent years, fertility specialists have also prescribed these medications as adjuncts for ovulation-induction treatments. The pros and cons of this approach will be discussed in later chapters.

On the surface it might appear paradoxical to use insulin-lowering medications to treat diabetics. However, type 2 diabetics actually have high insulin levels and a reduced ability to respond to insulin (i.e., insulin resistance). Many insulin-resistant women have Syndrome O because while certain tissues, such as muscle and fat, have become resistant to insulin's actions, their ovaries and HPO circle actually remain quite sensitive to insulin. More significantly, many women with Syndrome O have undiagnosed diabetes or a pre-diabetic problem called glucose intolerance. Good evidence indicates that women who focus on nutrition, activity, and stress reduction as part of their ongoing personal life-management strategies will gain safer, long-term insulin-lowering benefits for their fertility, pregnancies, and overall health.

WHEN THE MOON NEVER RISES: OVULATION DISRUPTION

Like the predictable phases of the moon, monthly menstrual cycles usually indicate that follicle growth and ovulation are occurring on a regular basis. However, as the ovaries become increasingly overwhelmed with insulin and androgens, ovulation disruption soon follows, often as early in life as adolescence. With each passing year, this problem intensifies if overnourishment, insulin overproduction, and ovarian confusion persist. Irregular and unpredictable patterns of menstrual bleeding usually means that ovulation is either taking place rarely (*oligoovulation*), or not at all (*anovulation*). A complete absence of menstrual cycles can also indicate anovulation and should be carefully evaluated by a women's health specialist. Medical conditions other than Syndrome O can cause this problem.

Ovulation disruption is one of the most common reasons for women to seek medical attention, and the underlying causes are commonly misdiagnosed, minimized, or ignored by the health-care community.

Ovulation disruption can cause heavy unpredictable vaginal bleeding or lighter and unremitting spotting. Fertility will always be compromised, yet undesired pregnancies may sometimes occur. Miscarriage is more common. Other important factors contributing to ovulation disruption include chronic stress, undernourishment, eating disorders, excess exercise, and certain medications. Thyroid, adrenal, and pituitary abnormalities will also cause ovulation disruption, as will early or premenopause. However, overnourishment and insulin overproduction—Syndrome O—are the most common disruptors of follicle growth and egg release.

In most instances of ovulation disruption, excess insulin and androgens inhibit the growth of a dominant, or winning, follicle. Rhythmic, pulsing signals of FSH and LH from the pituitary are also affected. Alternatively, a dominant follicle may grow during certain months, but enzymes required to thin the follicle wall and release the egg aren't properly activated. This may be due to direct insulin effects on enzymes and enzyme inhibitors within the follicle, or more global effects on the HPO circle causing inhibition of the LH surge.

For some women who present with pain, a large unruptured follicle can be seen as a fluid-filled cyst on ultrasound examination. Most of these cysts usually stop growing and eventually resorb without causing further symptoms. However, unresolved large follicular cysts can sometimes lead to ovarian torsion (twisting), cyst rupture, and internal bleeding—all potential surgical emergencies. Medical management of these emergencies is sometimes inadequate, yet surgical treatment is often too aggressive, leading to removal of an ovary and/or fallopian tube. In many instances, prompt evaluation by an experienced gynecologist is needed. If surgery is required, conservative organ-sparing surgery by laparoscopy is usually curative.

On a chronic basis, ovulation disruption will have a negative influence on the uterine lining, also called the *endometrium*. Chronic, yet inappropriate signals of androgens, estrogens, insulin, and insulin-like growth factors cause an abnormal transformation of the endometrium. Continuous estrogen and insulin exposure in the absence of progesterone can often lead to an important Syndrome O–related

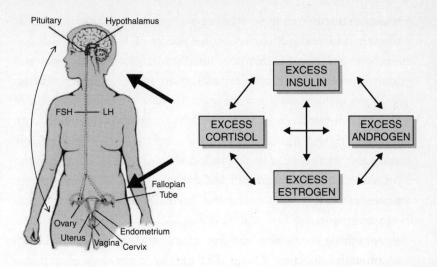

health hazard called *hyperplasia*. Certain types of hyperplasia are pre-cancerous and without appropriate treatment and monitoring, young women can develop endometrial cancer.

"I'm Lucky to Be Alive" is a title that screamed from a March 2000 issue of *Woman's Day.* Author Kerri Smith discussed how lucky she was to have survived endometrial cancer. At age thirty-seven, af-ter seeking care from several different doctors, she finally learned that her abnormal uterine bleeding was due to a relatively common form of uterine cancer. Abnormal growth of the uterine lining leading to cancer is a life-threatening risk for women like Kerri Smith, yet most other women are unaware of this Syndrome O–related danger. Her numerous poignant stories, published serially in the *Denver Post,* also described lifelong battles with insulin resistance, weight challenges, and polycystic ovaries.

All women with a diagnosis of polycystic ovaries and/or Syndrome O should be monitored for the possibility of en-dometrial hyperplasia or cancer, particularly if many months have passed with no menses or if chronic and unpredictable episodes of spotting and bleeding have occurred. Women who are taking progesterone on a regular basis, the contraceptive Depo-Provera, or oral contraceptive pills are at significantly less risk for developing endometrial hyperplasia or cancer. Other causes of irregular or abnormal bleeding include uterine polyps or fibroids, which can coexist with Syndrome O. Sensitive tests such as sonohysterography and hysteroscopy should be employed to diagnose and treat these problems.

Why do women who ovulate regularly have a much lower risk of endometrial hyperplasia or cancer, when compared to women with Syndrome O? During normal ovulation cycles, the ovaries reliably produce progesterone for twelve to fourteen days, which protects the endometrium from overgrowth and hyperplasia. The main purpose of progesterone is to prepare the endometrium for embryo implantatioon and pregnancy.

Progesterone is produced in large quantities by granulosa cells still attached to the ovulated follicle. The LH surge not only contributes to egg release at ovulation but also converts the ovulated follicle to a structure called the *corpus luteum,* or yellow body. High concentrations of LDL-cholesterol and related fatty acids in the corpus luteum cause the yellow color and two key enzymes are very active in converting LDL-cholesterol to progesterone. LH—luteinizing hormone—was originally named because it converts granulosa cells to progesterone-producing lutein cells.

Once a pregnancy occurs, the corpus luteum is maintained by placental *HCG—human chorionic gonadotropin.* HCG and LH are very similar hormone molecules, although HCG is longer acting and more stable. For years, HCG has been used as a medication to induce ovulation and help sustain an early pregnancy. Placental cells also contribute progesterone, but early pregnancy maintenance is still highly dependent on ovarian progesterone. Toward the end of the first trimester, the placenta takes over the major share of progesterone production and ovarian production diminishes.

When a pregnancy does not occur, the corpus luteum gradually stops functioning and progesterone production falls. In a normal menstrual cycle it is the drop in progesterone that induces sloughing of the endometrium and menstrual bleeding. This is a critical process, since it prevents the abnormal buildup of the uterine lining. The endometrium is the most actively remodeled tissue in the human body.

Soon after it is shed, the endometrium normally heals and regenerates in response to rising estrogen from newly emerging follicles. However, in a setting of ovulation disruption caused by Syndrome O, follicle growth may not occur in a subsequent cycle, causing prolonged and abnormal uterine bleeding.

The process of ovulation has worked well in humans, other animal species, and even in plants for millions of years. Syndrome O is a twentieth/twenty-first century problem. It is my firm belief that most Syndrome O women were born with the necessary genetic and organ machinery to ovulate on a regular basis. Sadly, the environment we all share has interfered with ovulation for millions of women around the world. Overnourishment, underactivity, and stress are the major co-conspirators. As you continue to tackle Syndrome O challenges, you will realize that honesty, determination, and freedom to make choices are your strong suits. Realigning your own environment so it best fits your genetic heritage can make all the difference for your fertility, pregnancy, and health.

KEY MOTIVATIONAL POINTS

- You started from a good egg and sperm. You were likely born with all of the genes necessary to be fertile and to lead a healthy and productive life.
- Your ovaries are part of the glandular internet, a fascinating hormonal system that allows communication between every organ in the body, including the brain.
- Follicle growth and ovulation are under the immediate control of hormonal cross-talk, which includes the brain's hypothalamus, the pituitary gland, and your ovaries—the hypothalamic-pituitary-ovarian (HPO) axis, or circle.
- Overnourishment and insulin overproduction commonly interfere with women's HPO circle, leading to the other Syndrome O problems of ovarian confusion and ovulation disruption.

- Certain lifestyle factors can significantly interfere with fertility, including consuming excessive amounts of sugar, starches, and funny fats, and stress inducers like the screen demons and poor sleep patterns. Personal efforts and strategies to focus on these factors in your life are an important first step in outsmarting Syndrome O.
- Ovarian confusion is the exaggerated production and distribution of vital androgens throughout the body. Excess androgen signals are further aggravated by the impact of insulin overproduction on the liver and adrenal glands.
- Ovulation disruption leads to common women's health problems—missed and irregular menstrual cycles, unpredictable and heavy bleeding, ovarian cysts, and infertility. Women with Syndrome O are at highest risk of developing precancerous or cancerous changes in the uterus compared to women who ovulate regularly. Ongoing medical surveillance is strongly advised.

THREE

THE INSULIN STORM: WHAT DOCTORS SHOULD BE TELLING YOU ABOUT OVERNOURISHMENT

THE "I" OF THE STORM

Inspiration and information will improve your life and enable you to achieve your goals. Is enhancing your fertility now, or in the future, a high priority for you? If so, you'll probably want to prepare your mind and body for a trouble-free pregnancy, followed by years of rewarding motherhood. Even if fertility is not currently a priority for you, healthfulness, vitality, and the impact of Syndrome O deserve your special attention. Consider saying to yourself: "I can have a better life. I can have a healthier life. I can have a fertile life. I can and must outsmart Syndrome O." After all, the "I" of the insulin storm is you.

It has taken many years for the medical community to gradually accept the reality that too much insulin can interfere with vital organ systems, including the heart, blood vessels, liver, muscle, and fat tissue. Dr. Gerald Reaven is widely credited with expanding this viewpoint regarding chronic insulin overproduction, also known as *hyperinsulinemia* (*hyper* = high, *emia* = in the blood, i.e. "high insulin in the blood").

In 1988, when delivering the highly revered Banting address to the American Diabetes Association, Dr. Reaven first introduced Syndrome X. He described Syndrome X as a *whole body phenomenon of insulin resistance and insulin overproduction,* leading to diverse health problems. The major premise of Syndrome X is that a large percentage of the body's cells do not respond efficiently to insulin. Although insulin has several important functions along the glandular internet, its most immediate life-preserving job is to shuttle glucose fuel into cells. Without a constant source of glucose, most cells would die. If a normal amount of insulin inefficiently performs this life-giving task, the glandular internet quickly informs the pancreas to produce more insulin. Cells that do not respond to insulin effectively are described as *insulin resistant.*

Muscle cells are major users of glucose and underused muscle tissue is very prone to being insulin resistant. Even in this circumstance, muscle tissue strongly requires glucose. To meet this demand, additional insulin must be pumped from the pancreas through the blood stream to help the muscle's metabolic needs. As the body's resistance to insulin worsens, insulin overproduction becomes more pronounced. Dr. Reaven and other experts refer to this as "compensatory hyperinsulinemia." *Overnourishment* both incites and exacerbates insulin resistance and further promotes chronic insulin overproduction.

Not all organs in the body require or desire extra insulin. When the glandular internet is overburdened with insulin, major Syndrome X

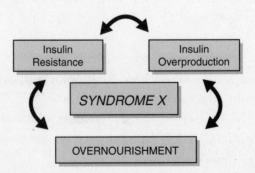

pathways to disease are now well defined—*cardiovascular disease* and *metabolic disease.* Once a vicious cycle of insulin overproduction is under way, metabolic disease contributes to cardiovascular disease through excess circulating fats and cholesterol, and their atherosclerotic effects on blood vessels in the heart and throughout the body. Cardiovascular disease, by way of decreased activity and exercise intolerance, can worsen metabolic disease. About half of all American adults—men and women—are affected in some way by the Syndrome X cascade of insulin overproduction. Even more concerning is the knowledge that a high percentage of American children and teenagers have already developed significant insulin resistance problems such as obesity and type 2 diabetes.

The roots of insulin resistance and Syndrome X appear quite similar to the lifestyle factors that were described in chapter 2—the wrong quality and quantity of food, too much unburned sugar calories, funny fats, too much stress, and too little activity. A hereditary predisposition toward a thrifty, famine-surviving metabolism further aggravates the problem. We should be careful to distinguish the concept of a genetic predisposition from that of an actual genetic disease. In most instances, neither Syndrome X nor Syndrome O are genetic diseases. Since insulin resistance appears to affect people from virtually every race and ethnic heritage in the world, these syndromes actually reflect a tendency of our genes to adapt and react to changes in the environment as they see fit.

Scientists, physicians, and many other health professionals have gradually put together the pieces of the glandular internet puzzle as it

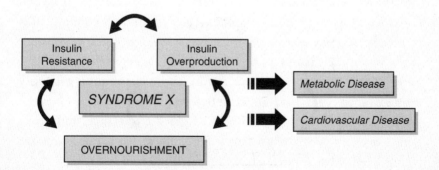

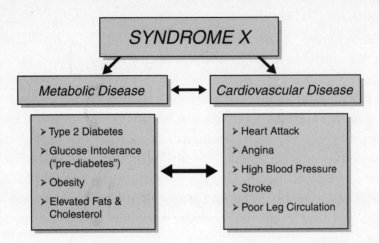

applies specifically to women. It is estimated that 5 to 10 million young women in the United States have significant reproductive health consequences related to insulin overproduction. For most women who are affected, reproductive problems lead them to seek medical advice and treatment.

A large focus of my work and philosophical approach has been to educate and motivate women about the influence of insulin overproduction upon their fertility and pregnancy health. Since the impact of insulin overproduction is so different for women as compared to men, I developed the concept of Syndrome O to help women better recognize vital connections between their metabolism and reproductive system.

Both Syndrome O and Syndrome X invoke themes of insulin overproduction, as a result of chronic overnourishment and insulin resistance. However, for most women, the Syndrome X consequences of metabolic and cardiovascular disease have not become as apparent as the Syndrome O impact upon fertility and the reproductive system. Nevertheless, in my practice, we test for and will commonly identify many women who have overt and severe insulin overproduction, profound lipid abnormalities, impaired glucose tolerance, and actual type 2 diabetes. Many physicians still believe that it is impossible for young women to harbor such abnormal blood values.

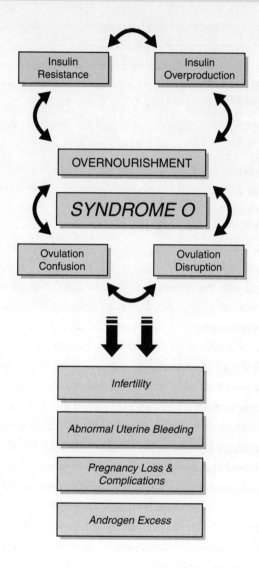

GETTING FAT: LET'S DEFINE OVERNOURISHMENT

My computer's spellchecker is unhappy with the word *overnourish-ment*, which doesn't appear in its dictionary. Yet it has no problem with the word *undernourishment*. Historically, and even in many parts of the world today, mankind has suffered from undernourishment.

Hundreds of generations of humans throughout the world evolved metabolic and reproductive systems to withstand undernourishment. However, we now have another global food-related problem.

Scientifically, in order for the body to maintain a state of balance, or *homeostasis* (or, as Isaac Newton said, for every action there is an equal and opposite reaction), and adapt to long periods of undernourishment, occasional episodes of overnourishment were actually beneficial for human survival. Traditions of feasting to celebrate special holidays or events have roots in virtually every culture and ethnic heritage around the world.

Just as automobile engines require hydrocarbon-based fuels for energy, living cells universally require glucose, a relatively simple carbon-hydrogen combination (or *carbohydrate*). And just as an average car can travel about twenty miles with one gallon of gasoline, the average human can stay alive for about two hours with the energy derived from metabolizing only *one ounce* of glucose. Theoretically, just twelve ounces of glucose (which can be found in about seven bottles of soda), would suffice to maintain twenty-four hours of human life. It is truly amazing how energy-efficient the human body can be!

Our modern carbohydrate requirements are a hot topic right now, with various nutritional gurus advocating all sorts of combinations of carbohydrate, fat, and protein in our diet. Even the U.S. government has gotten into the game, suggesting that every American citizen would benefit from a daily food pyramid diet containing mostly carbohydrates (i.e., six to eleven servings from the bread, cereal, rice, and pasta group, *and* five to nine servings of fruits and vegetables), and relatively little dairy (two to three servings) or meat, eggs, fish, and poultry (two to three servings). It is hard to know if each and every citizen in the entire United States, from every ethnic heritage, and with varying degrees of insulin resistance, is well served by these guidelines (www.health.gov/dietaryguidelines). It is also interesting to speculate as to whether our nation would be healthier if most people actually followed these guidelines.

Protein and fats are also biological hydrocarbons and can be used indirectly as energy sources if insufficient glucose is available. Protein, when digested and broken down to its amino acid building blocks, provides about the same energy per unit weight as glucose. Fat is much more efficient, however, providing more than twice the amount of energy as carbohydrate or protein. Theoretically, an average-size individual could stay alive for an entire day with the energy derived from just five ounces of either animal or vegetable fat.

The energy units of the three macronutrients—carbohydrate, protein, and fat—are called *calories.* One gram of carbohydrate or protein provides 4 calories; a gram of fat yields 9 calories. The combinations of carbohydrate, protein, and fat determine the complete caloric content of any particular food. Energy consumption is not the only purpose for macronutrients, since these food components are also required to rebuild cells and tissues. Every cell in the body is constantly producing new enzymes and cellular components, requiring essential carbohydrates, fatty acids, and amino acids.

According to Isaac Newton's laws of physics, every morsel of ingested food must be accounted for, whether it is burned for energy, stored for future energy use, incorporated into essential cells and tissues, or excreted as waste. Our bodies have two principal ways to store excess calories: first as glycogen (long molecules of glucose resembling connected paper-doll cutouts); or second as fat (we all know what fat looks like). Glycogen can be stored in the muscle or the liver, and it provides just a few hours of extra energy during fasts or exertion. Athletes will commonly carb-load the day before a big competition so as to have their glycogen stores maximally filled.

Biochemists have names for every metabolic event, and *lipogenesis* is the name given to fat production and storage. Chronic and persistent fat storage is the essence of overnourishment, since fat can deposit itself just about everywhere. Most humans have been blessed with very efficient lipogenic enzymes, capable of converting excess nonutilized dietary sugars and fats into stored body fat. Central fat deposits around the midline, the so-called apple shape, have been commonly linked to insulin resistance and metabolic and cardiovascular diseases. Excess fat can also make its way into the muscle and liver, making the metabolic situation even more catastrophic.

Overnourishment does not just mean "overeating." It more precisely defines a state of ingesting more food calories than the body requires, based on activity levels and caloric burn rate. A pound of fat contains about 3,500 calories, which suggests that if an individual is "overnourished" by about 120 calories per day (i.e., about equal to one slice of bread), she could easily gain one pound each month, or about twelve pounds per year. A chronic and continuous pattern of weight gain usually implies chronic overnourishment. So, if that same individual who was overnourished by 120 calories per day decides to increase her activity by committing to a daily thirty-minute brisk walk, it is likely that her weight gain will rapidly stop. Many women tell me that they "just keep gaining weight" no matter how little they eat or how much they exercise. This simply does not fit with Newton's laws of physics.

Thinner individuals are not immune from insulin overproduction and overnourishment. Although ingested calories may not be absorbed from the intestines as readily or incorporated into fat tissue as efficiently, thin individuals can still suffer the metabolic, cardiovascular, and reproductive consequences of insulin overproduction. Thin women can also have Syndrome O, probably due to having reproductive organs that have a particularly exquisite inherited sensitivity to insulin. Although weight loss is not particularly beneficial *per se,* thin women with Syndrome O can also benefit greatly from insulin-reducing strategies designed to increase muscle mass and reduce excess carbohydrates in their diet.

Body Mass Index and Overnourishment

Most women think they have a good estimate of their ideal body weight. However, the *body mass index* (BMI) is commonly used to provide an objective number based on height and weight. The arithmetic formula for BMI is weight in kilograms divided twice by height in meters (i.e. BMI $= kg/m^2$). For people who like to calculate such things, it is necessary to convert your height from inches into meters (one inch $= 0.0254$ meters) and your weight from pounds into kilograms (1 pound = .454 kilogram). There are also readily available pre-calculated charts to determine your BMI, making the calculations unnecessary. BMI determinations apply equally to women or men. By way of example, an individual who is 5 feet 2 inches and weighs 131 pounds has a BMI of 24, which is considered normal. At 153 pounds, an individual of the same height has a BMI of 28 (considered overweight); at 180 pounds the BMI is 33 (considered obese).

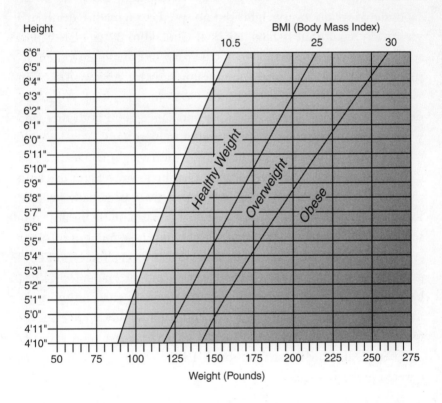

- Being overweight or obese may reduce a woman's fertility. When pregnancy is achieved, excessive weight increases risks associated with pregnancy.

- Weight loss may improve fertility and pregnancy outcome.

American Society for Reproductive Medicine, 2001

A high BMI is a significant risk factor for premature death. In a 1999 landmark article published in the *New England Journal of Medicine,* a group of epidemiologists from the American Cancer Society studied the impact of high BMI upon mortality. Their research was done in a prospective fashion (i.e., before the event), which is considered the most powerful way to assess outcomes in clinical science. For women who never smoked, the lowest risk of premature death occurred when the BMI was 19 to 22. Fortunately, a BMI up to 27 (considered mildly overweight) did not predict premature death in a statistically significant fashion. As BMI climbed to 32 or higher, premature death rates climbed 50 to 150 percent for Caucasian women, although they were not quite so ominously high for African-American women (about 20 percent increase). Common causes of premature death included cardiovascular disease and cancer, and both men and women were affected by the relationship to high BMI.

Most American adults are now either overweight (BMI of 25 to 29) or obese (BMI of 30 and above). Despite knowing and teaching the facts about overnourishment to my patients, I personally struggle to maintain my BMI between 28 and 30. I don't relish the health consequences proven to be associated with obesity. Like millions of other Americans, I am tempted by less-than-perfect food choices and burdened by sedentary hours of stressful sitting and screen demons. I feel best when I eat fewer calories and carbohydrates than my government recommends, avoid trans fats, and walk briskly an average of five to six hours each week. This has helped me maintain a steady number on the BMI chart, although I keep striving to achieve the coveted normal range.

PLENTY OF INSULIN: WHY DIABETES?

Diabetes is a scary word to many people, especially if they've witnessed the distressing consequences of the disease suffered by friends or loved ones. In its most chronic and severe form, diabetes directly promotes vascular changes in the eyes, kidneys, legs and feet, and heart. A major portion of our precious health-care resources is devoted to the ravages of diabetes-induced blindness, kidney failure, dialysis, renal transplants, limb amputations, wound care, and rehabilitation. The toll of human suffering related to diabetes is high. Increased efforts devoted to prevention and education would have likely helped many affected people.

Current statistics indicate that about one in fifteen Americans have diabetes, and countless others have the prediabetic state known as *glucose intolerance*. For the large majority of diabetic and prediabetic individuals, insulin resistance is the inciting cause, along with chronic overnourishment and obesity. Women are much more likely than men to confront diabetes at an earlier age, since they often face issues affecting their fertility, menstrual cycles, and pregnancy well-being. Volumes have been written about diabetes of pregnancy, also known as *gestational diabetes*. All pregnant women are now screened for gestational diabetes, since the impact on the developing fetus includes birth defects, metabolic derangements, stillbirth, and abnormal growth.

A new diagnosis of diabetes or prediabetes often sends a vital message to young women urging immediate changes in life management prior to fertility care and pregnancy. Important data indicate that a high number of Syndrome O women have undiagnosed diabetes or prediabetes and could be embarking on a dangerous pregnancy without the benefit of preconception care. It has become routine in my medical practice to test all women with Syndrome O for diabetes or glucose intolerance prior to starting fertility care. Although some practitioners advocate screening with just a simple fasting blood glucose level, we strongly recommend the more sensitive two-hour glucose tolerance test. This test challenges the body with a relatively small 300 calorie oral sugar load, with the expectation that insulin is able to maintain the blood glucose level in a normal range. If the body is resistant to insulin action, the blood glucose may remain elevated after two hours, indicating type 2 diabetes. Fortunately, most Syndrome O women do not yet have overt diabetes.

Why does diabetes develop in some women but not in others? The answer likely lies in the severity of each woman's insulin resistance and the degree of insulin overproduction required to meet the body's ongoing metabolic needs. Insulin is produced by one organ—the *pancreas*—and by one specialized type of cell within the pancreas—the *beta cells*. The beta cells are genetically programmed to produce and secrete insulin when glucose enters the bloodstream after eating. In a person who is not insulin-resistant, a relatively small amount of insulin is required to shuttle glucose into the tissues. For someone who is insulin-resistant, the pancreas is prodded to produce ever-increasing quantities of insulin immediately after food is absorbed into the bloodstream. As would be predicted, the degree of insulin over-production is highly dependent on the size of the meal, the makeup of the meal (i.e., proportion of carbohydrates, protein, and fat), and the extent of insulin resistance throughout the body. In diabetic in-dividuals—of whom there are 16 million or more in the United States—the pancreas cannot keep up with the demand for insulin fol-lowing meals. Without enough insulin, blood glucose levels rise. High glucose levels in the bloodstream that persist while fasting, or more than two hours after a meal, are the hallmark of diabetes.

Symptoms of undiagnosed diabetes, or even glucose intolerance, can include chronic and worsening fatigue, particularly following meals; constant thirst; frequent urination; blurred vision; weight loss without trying to lose weight; and frequent infections, such as blad-der and vaginal yeast infections. Many women with Syndrome O complain of constant cravings for sweets and other carbohydrates, suggesting that they have inefficient transport of glucose to their vi-tal organs. Syndrome O women frequently report a strong family his-tory of diabetes, heart disease, and obesity. Thus, thrifty metabolic genes tend to be inherited, and these highly evolved genes clearly clash with an environment promoting easy food access, low activity levels, and high stress. The pancreas hardly ever starts out diseased in most instances of type 2 diabetes. Sadly, more and more children and adolescents are now diagnosed with type 2 diabetes, suggesting that the struggle between genetics and environmental factors is worsening.

Researchers have found that a problem known as *beta cell dysfunc-tion* profoundly interferes with insulin production by the pancreas. In combination with insulin resistance throughout the body, worsening beta cell dysfunction both contributes to and exacerbates type 2 diabetes. Since the pancreas and its insulin-producing beta cells are part of the glandular internet, it is not surprising that chronic imbalances in metabolism worsen the predicament. Exposure to high glucose, elevated levels of fatty acids and certain inflammatory hormones called cytokines all worsen beta cell function. Reduction of glucose load and fatty acid levels appear to help beta cell function. Beta cell dysfunction may be analogous to certain cellular changes seen in the ovaries, since immediate changes in metabolism, overnourishment, and insulin overproduction must be instituted to reverse the abnormalities.

LOCKING THE BARN

Great as our interest is in the cure of disease, the truly inspiring word of modern medicine is not cure but prevention. It is well to recover the horse stolen from the unlocked barn—if you can. It is proverbially better to lock the barn before the horse is stolen.

How do these banalities apply to the problem of the pancreas and diabetes? Very tangibly, I believe. It is a well-recognized clinical observation that the majority of diabetic subjects were very overweight—downright fat, to speak brusquely—before they became obviously diabetic. This may mean in some cases that there were inherited defects of metabolism or imbalances of endocrine glands other than the pancreas. But it is more likely to mean that the fat person was fat because he or she ate too much food.

The terse phrase, "Food makes Fat"—coined, I believe, by Miss Fanny Hurst after painful personal tests of its truth—should become a classic. As a corollary only a degree less forceful, one might epitomize the pancreas situation in the paraphrase, Food makes Diabetes.

It is true that food does not always make fat. It is even more true that not all fat people become diabetics. But epigrams are not subjects for inquisitorial dissection. Suffice it that no person who did not ingest more food than his body consumed ever became fat; and that few persons who had not habitually imposed on their digestive organs more food than was requisite to bodily needs ever became diabetics. Usually, but not always, the excess food is registered as accumulated fat, before the pancreatic revolt makes itself manifest in shortage of insulin and consequent rise of blood sugar.

Again the good old moral bobs up. Again, we need not labor it. In more than the conventional sense, this is a case where he who runs may read. For that matter, it is a case where running—good, active running—will do more good than any amount of reading.★

★Excerpt from *Your Glands and You,* Henry Smith Williams, M.D., 1936.

The incidence of type 2 diabetes in the United States appears to have increased over 6,000 percent in the past seventy years. This strongly suggests that problems like Syndromes X and O are all phenomena of modern living. If you believe you might have diabetes, or the pre-diabetic problem of glucose intolerance, you are urged to seek immediate evaluation and treatment. It is well beyond the scope of this book to provide specifics regarding diabetes care, yet it is the mission of this book to contribute to education and diabetes prevention. Many believe that homespun wisdom can often serve as the best medicine, and such advice related to diabetes has existed for many years.

Insulin and Your Liver: A Stab at the Heart

To sound the alarm even louder, high BMI, type 2 diabetes, and insulin resistance are major contributors to cardiovascular disease. It is well established that people with type 2 diabetes have a 100 to 200 percent increased chance of dying from cardiovascular disease when compared with the nondiabetic population. The liver is the critical organ within the glandular internet connecting chaotic metabolism with cardiovascular disease. By recognizing states of both undernourishment and overnourishment, the liver responds in a genetically programmed fashion. Through a detailed and fascinating array of calorie-manipulating enzymes, the liver helps maintain metabolic equilibrium (*homeostasis*) and a steady supply of glucose fuel for the body's ongoing survival.

Remembering that mild to severe undernourishment was the norm in the history of mankind, humans evolved specialized enzymes to ward off starvation until the next meal arrived. Most significant are fat-burning, or *lipolysis,* enzymes, capable of breaking down both stored and ingested fat. An ounce of stored fat will supply about 270 calories of usable energy, enough for hunting, fishing, or gardening for one to two hours. If fat burning is prolonged for days, chemical by-products called *ketone bodies* will be produced, which suppress a person's appetite until food can be caught or harvested.

If undernourishment becomes more severe, on the level of prolonged starvation, the body can also utilize its own muscle protein as fuel. Amino acids, the basic building blocks of protein, are converted by liver enzymes into glucose through a process called *gluconeogenesis.* Although popular diets advocating high protein intake can initially trick the body into burning fat and protein, excess ingested calories from this approach will most certainly be converted to glucose and stored as fat. Furthermore, just a tad of "cheating" by eating some excess unburned carbohydrates will quickly halt the fat-burning enzymes and actually accelerate fat storage.

Insulin overproduction was hardly a concern while the liver was working hard to sustain life during times of undernourishment. The pancreatic beta cells only needed to produce and secrete tiny quantities of insulin into the bloodstream to shuttle glucose fuel to the body's tissues. In addition, so-called counter-regulatory hormones such as glucagon (from the pancreas), growth hormone (from the pituitary), and cortisol (from the adrenals) helped keep blood sugar levels stable. Humans from all ethnic backgrounds seem to share this evolutionary imperative to require low quantities of ingested food for survival, as well as reproduction.

When food did arrive to our ancestors, it was usually in the form of fresh, lean meat, fish, or wild grains, fruits, and vegetables. Those were really the only choices of food for all of mankind, virtually everywhere on the planet. Wild game meat contains very low quantities of saturated fat, whereas fish and other seafood contain special fats of the omega-3 varieties. Grain, fruits, and vegetables provided mostly carbohydrates, but with low density and low glycemic indices. Primitive man probably also learned about comfort calories, such as those derived from fermented grains or cocoa beans, or probably from fatty organs such as brain and liver.

Overeating and overnourishment were hardly seen, but during times when food was more plentiful, the liver did its job to efficiently store excess ingested calories. Thus, the liver has the major task of converting glucose and fatty acids to lipids, the process called *lipogenesis*. In addition, the liver has the important task of producing cholesterol, a backbone molecule for vital ovarian and adrenal hormones.

Overnourishment dramatically shifts the liver to an active lipogenic and cholesterol-producing organ. If you inherited genes from ancestors who had very efficient lipogenic enzymes, and if you are overnourished, you will likely have high levels of triglycerides (i.e. fats) and/or cholesterol circulating in your bloodstream. Insulin overproduction and diabetes worsen the situation. Since recently eaten fats can temporarily raise both triglyceride and cholesterol levels, it is recommended that blood lipid levels be checked during a fasting state. High triglyceride and LDL-cholesterol levels lead to life-

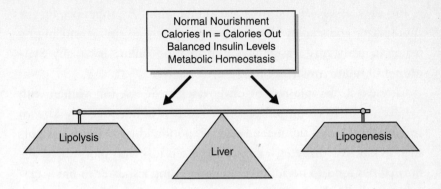

threatening plaque deposits in major arteries, including those that supply blood to the heart.

Overnourishment increases the availability of free fatty acids to the liver for lipogenesis, while free fatty acids worsen pancreatic beta cell function and insulin resistance throughout the body. Most women with Syndrome O have elevated levels of fasting triglycerides and cholesterol. Cardiologists have formulas for calculating cardiovascular risk based on triglyceride and cholesterol levels.

Insulin sends other important signals to the liver that affect cardiovascular risk, through the enhanced production of proteins that promote blood clotting. Under normal circumstances, the liver synthesizes an array of proteins that regulate when and where the blood will clot, and the proper timing for blood clots to be removed. Insulin overproduction is strongly associated with an abnormally high prothrombotic tendency, leading to an additional risk factor for thrombotic

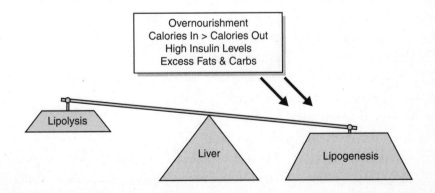

events such as stroke and myocardial infarction. A propensity for inappropriate and excess blood clotting is likely to be a contributing factor to early miscarriage and implantation failure for many Syndrome O women who are trying to conceive.

The exact elevated risk of cardiovascular disease for women with Syndrome O as compared to other women is not precisely known and will likely vary significantly between individuals. Multiple factors such as obesity, diabetes, chronic hypertension, and blood lipid abnormalities tend to be additive when assessing risk later in life. Cigarette smoking dramatically worsens the risk. Fortunately, younger women are not frequently diagnosed with stroke, angina, or myocardial infarction, but most underlying blood vessel disease can remain silent for many years. In some instances, lipid-lowering drugs are advocated to lower the long-term cardiovascular risk, although these medications are absolutely contraindicated for women who are trying to get pregnant. Lipid-lowering drugs act by diminishing the action of lipogenic enzymes in the liver, many of which are directly stimulated by insulin. Insulin-lowering nutritional and activity strategies can have the same benefit.

Can liver action be improved by modifications in nutrition and activity? As part of the glandular internet, the liver can quickly adjust to metabolic change, especially if fat burning (lipolysis) is favored and fat creation (lipogenesis) is diminished. The key is eliminating overnourishment from your body and vocabulary and identifying an intelligent day-to-day balance of carbohydrate, protein, fats, *and* muscular activ-

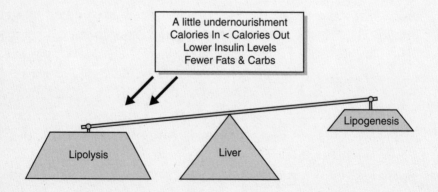

ity. No one is commanding you to be overnourished! A plan of life management, along with careful evaluation and treatment from your physician, is a great two-prong approach

BAND-AID BUT NOT A CURE: A FEW WORDS ABOUT BIRTH CONTROL PILLS

No medicine has been invented yet to cure Syndrome O, nor the underlying problems of overnourishment and insulin overproduction. However, birth control pills (BCPs) can restore a more regular menstrual pattern and will often help women avoid difficult episodes of heavy, unstoppable bleeding. Nevertheless, it is critical to understand that BCPs will neither reverse nor cure the metabolic and fertility challenges caused by Syndrome O.

BCPs may be a helpful therapeutic option to consider if you are currently trying to outsmart the metabolic aspects of Syndrome O, yet are not interested in getting pregnant. Modern BCPs contain conservative doses of synthetic estrogens and progestins, designed to suppress production of FSH and LH hormones from the pituitary gland. As a result, FSH stimulation of ovarian follicles and LH stimulation of androgen production is dramatically reduced, leading to very effective blockage of follicle growth. A potential benefit for some women is the dramatic reduction in circulating ovarian androgens in the bloodstream, although others complain of decreased libido possibly as a result of lowered androgen levels. For women with Syndrome O, the progestin component of the BCP provides much needed hormone protection for the endometrial lining of the uterus. However, if your doctor is suspicious of a precancerous change in the endometrium, an excessively thick uterine lining, or polyps, these possibilities must be evaluated before you start taking BCPs.

On a longer-term basis, BCPs can exert some desired effects on production of certain sponge proteins by the liver. As an example, estrogen stimulates the liver to produce extra sex hormone binding globulin (SHBG), a protein that protects the skin, hair follicles, and sebaceous glands from excessive androgens. Syndrome O women tend to have low levels of SHBG, because high insulin tells the liver to produce less SHBG. Thus, BCPs can have a double benefit for Syndrome O women who suffer with acne or have excess hair growth throughout the body (hirsutism). By reducing ovarian androgens and increasing SHBG, there will likely be much less free, or bioactive, androgens in the bloodstream. After a number of months, BCPs can exert some improvements in complexion and undesired hair growth.

There is one relatively rare yet significant complication of BCPs. An increased incidence of thromboembolic events will be seen in certain BCP users, and this may be due to a combination of events— a genetic predisposition related to certain clotting proteins, along with the production of extra clotting proteins induced by BCP use. Uncorrected insulin overproduction, as well as type 2 diabetes, can worsen the propensity for blood clot formation, as previously discussed. Cigarette smoking compounds the clotting risk dramatically. Although controversial, some researchers have found that certain progestin hormones, including those found in BCPs, can worsen insulin resistance, setting up a potential vicious cycle for Syndrome O women who are trying to control their insulin levels. An informed decision to use BCPs, particularly for women with Syndrome O, requires the knowledge and recommendations of a skilled health provider. This same recommendation applies to newer combination hormone patch contraceptives and injections of long-acting progestins, like Depo-Provera.

Short-term BCP use has some significant advantages for women who are pursuing fertility treatments, and we use BCPs in our practice as a way to efficiently implement ovulation-inducing medications. It is likely that just one month of BCPs can help improve the ovarian and uterine environment prior to treatment. Of course, we also urge simultaneous and preemptive nonpharmacologic lifestyle changes for Syndrome O women that are designed to improve metabolism and lower insulin levels. Important suggestions for lifestyle changes are addressed in greater detail in chapters 8 and 9.

Working to Calm the Insulin Storm: Key Motivational Points

- Overnourishment and insulin overproduction affect men and women differently. Unlike Syndrome X, Syndrome O encompasses the metabolic and fertility consequences of excess insulin that are unique to women.
- Insulin resistance and insulin overproduction go hand in hand. It is hard to know which starts first, although overnourishment is probably the underlying cause. When cells in the body become resistant to insulin's action, the pancreas must work harder to compensate. As a result, extra insulin is produced, affecting the entire body in many different ways.
- Syndrome O is not a genetic disease, and it is unlikely that any specific abnormal genes will be identified. More likely, millions of women from around the world have inherited a superior set of genes that allowed survival of their ancestors during famine and successful reproduction in a setting of low insulin levels.
- With thrifty genes as the basis for our ancestors' survival, it is easy for Americans to become fat. Most people in our country—including men, women, and children—are overnourished, accounting for our current epidemic of obesity. Body mass index (BMI) provides a score to assess nourishment state, taking into account an individual's height and weight.
- Overnourishment is simply defined as ingesting more calories than your body requires, taking activity levels (or lack thereof) into account. Unlike an automobile that only functions with gas in the tank, humans have evolved elegant enzyme systems for *lipolysis,* burning fat when calories are scarce, and *lipogenesis,* producing and storing fat when extra calories are eaten.

- One in fifteen Americans has type 2 diabetes, which results when insulin resistance outstrips the ability of the pancreas to keep up with the body's insulin requirements. Ironically, insulin overproduction is still present in most cases of type 2 diabetes. The incidence of diabetes has increased 6,000 percent since the 1930s, suggesting that our environment and lifestyle are major factors.

- All women with Syndrome O should be screened for diabetes and glucose intolerance, a pre-diabetic state. Since insulin overproduction and diabetes greatly enhances cardiovascular risk, women need to be informed about current and future risk of stroke and heart disease.

- The liver is a pivotal organ in determining fat and cholesterol production. Many enzyme steps promoting lipogenesis are controlled by insulin, with excess insulin contributing to high triglyceride and LDL-cholesterol values. The balance between lipogenesis and lipolysis can be modified dramatically through insulin-lowering strategies.

- Insulin overproduction can worsen the predisposition for thrombosis, further contributing to stroke and myocardial infarction later in life. Women with Syndrome O are at higher risk for miscarriage, possibly due to a higher thrombosis tendency at the site of pregnancy implantation in the uterus.

- Birth control pills have some advantages for women with Syndrome O. However, each woman must be assessed individually before taking BCPs, with the pros and cons carefully delineated. BCPs will not cure Syndrome O, nor will other hormonal contraceptives, such as the birth control patch or injections of Depo-Provera.

FOUR

SWEET CONCEPTIONS:
THE DECISION TO START A FAMILY

When a couple makes the monumental decision to start a family, they are blessed with a life goal that is shared and special. Often it is associated with butterflies-in-the-stomach anticipation and a little apprehension. Most couples assume that conceiving a child will happen naturally and seamlessly. Sadly, one in eight couples in the United States who are actively working toward a pregnancy will be incorrect in that assumption. During their entire reproductive years, about one in three couples will have trouble either conceiving or carrying a successful pregnancy. According to the National Institutes of Health, this translates into about 5 million couples per year in the United States who actively face ongoing challenges with their fertility.

It is the responsibility of physicians who care for reproductive-age men and women to be aware of the high prevalence of infertility in our society and to make appropriate judgments in evaluation, treatment, and referrals. Likewise, couples that are having trouble conceiving should not suffer in silence or retreat into denial. Unfortunately, many couples are embarrassed and scared about their fertility problems and may delay seeking care for months or years. This is true even when there are some great fertility experts and clinics right in their own backyard. Although access to good care can sometimes be geographically and/or financially problematic for many couples, my motto remains: "If you ask enough questions, you'll eventually get some good answers."

With a new wave of consumerism and a vast array of alternative medicine options available, both information overload and confusion are common. For a problem as widespread as infertility, it is no surprise that hundreds of books have been published describing the wonders of high-tech fertility treatments. Identifying good information on the Internet compounds the problem. With a natural bias toward marketing, many informational Web sites tend to stress the revenue-generating treatment portions of fertility care, rather than the virtues of careful and detailed medical evaluation. I believe this phenomenon is true whether the sponsoring clinics are private, hospital affiliated, or university-based.

Based on observations in our practice and informal surveys from colleagues, Syndrome O likely causes 20 to 25 percent of female factor infertility cases. Yet, there is a paucity of good information specifically written for Syndrome O women who are seeking fertility care and a healthy pregnancy. Syndrome O may also be a significant factor in 20 percent or more of first trimester miscarriages, which total about one million per year in the United States. It is very clear that Syndrome O women have extremely high rates of infertility and pregnancy loss.

The goals for this section of *Healing Syndrome O* are to provide comprehensive guidelines tailored to the needs of Syndrome O women who want to conceive and carry a healthy pregnancy. The information has its roots in evidence-based medicine, corroborated by insightful observations made in my practice of reproductive endocrinology and infertility. It is not intended to be a substitution for seeking necessary care and evaluation from your doctors. As in any field of medicine, not all doctors agree on the interpretation of medical studies, or on the applicability of those studies to clinical practice.

Whether in academic, hospital-based, or private practice centers, you should feel confident that your physicians are constantly striving to enhance the effectiveness of your fertility care. Our ethical mission is to try our best to do the right thing for every patient and to provide education and information at each step.

Leave No Stone Unturned

When a couple garners the courage to first seek advice from a fertility specialist, they usually have many questions and concerns. Common questions are:

- What is wrong with me (us)?
- What are our chances of getting pregnant?
- Will tests and treatments be painful?
- If I use fertility drugs, will I have a multiple pregnancy?
- How much will this cost?
- What if treatments don't work?

A comprehensive initial evaluation and pretreatment consultation should take all of these vital questions into account, along with a host of others. Although specific answers may not be known until some careful detective work is carried out, an honest assessment of the time and cost required should be provided from the outset.

It truly takes a caring team approach to make a baby. During a couple's first visit to our practice we provide separate and private detailed consultations with the doctor, a nurse or nurse practitioner experienced in the field, and a health insurance/financial specialist. Since so much information is provided at this first visit, new patients are asked to return for a second visit so that a thorough exam and ultrasound can be carried out. In an efficient manner, requisite blood labs and other tests can be ordered and the results interpreted.

How do we formulate the diagnosis of Syndrome O? Although for teaching purposes I have simplified Syndrome O into the triad of *overnourishment, ovarian confusion,* and *ovulation disruption,* my medical investigation requires obtaining concrete objective information from each patient. With that, a pattern emerges that helps me develop an impression and diagnosis. I believe that Syndrome O can be accurately diagnosed 90 percent of the time following a detailed consultation. Physical examination, ultrasound evaluation, and laboratory studies help confirm or refute the initial impression and may also uncover other underlying problems. Despite the yearning a couple may have to become pregnant, there are no shortcuts in this process. Incomplete and shoddy evaluations or an inappropriate rush to treatment can often lead to wasted time, money, and lost opportunities for a successful pregnancy.

Although doctors are often looking for a single specific diagnosis to explain a couple's problem, the reasons behind infertility are not always cut-and-dry. Any physician who provides evaluation or treatment services to infertile couples should be on the watch for other contributing factors. Too often, women are handed prescriptions for fertility medicines like clomiphene or gonadotropins without the benefit of closer scrutiny of other potential pregnancy roadblocks. Unfortunately, Syndrome O women and their loving partners are not immune from other common problems, such as male factor infertility, fallopian tube disease, pelvic adhesions, uterine polyps, and fibroids. Treatment options could vary significantly when these additional factors are identified. Endometriosis can also be a significant factor for many women suffering from infertility, although that disease tends to be found less frequently in women with Syndrome O.

Our clinical staff utilizes a detailed checklist so we don't overlook Syndrome O or any other potential fertility problems. Consider using the question list entitled "Could I Have Syndrome O?" in chapter 1 to enhance the value of your consultations and evaluation. The following are additional questions you might wish to think about.

- **What is the male partner's sperm count and quality?**
  Women's bodies aren't the only factor in fertility. It is always necessary to evaluate the male partner in order to check for

less than optimal semen quality. A semen analysis showing a normal sperm count, motility, and morphology (appearance) usually rules out a significant male problem. A sample for semen analysis should be collected after forty-eight to seventy-two hours of abstinence from ejaculation, and should be evaluated promptly by a certified laboratory. If the parameters are consistently below the norm, we strongly recommend referral to a urologist who specializes in male infertility problems. An accurate diagnosis must be made before instituting treatments. Some couples, based on sperm problems alone, are better served by *in vitro* fertilization (IVF), which is described in detail in chapter 5.

Relatively mild male problems can include a varicocele (a hemorrhoid-like growth of a vein in the scrotum), regular exposure to high-temperature environments (for example, a factory or even a hot tub), and exposure to certain toxins (like pesticides). More severe problems include congenital abnormalities of the testes or vas deferens (a tube carrying sperm from the testes), undescended testicles, tumors, and certain genetic or chromosome abnormalities. Diabetes can cause neurological problems, erectile dysfunction, and retrograde (backward) ejaculation. Each problem needs to be evaluated individually. On many occasions, even men who have been diagnosed with azoospermia—a complete absence of sperm in the semen—*can* father children. We continue to see couples on a frequent basis that believed for years they could not have children due to the husband's absence of sperm. A minor outpatient procedure to aspirate or biopsy a small portion of the testes can completely change the fertility prognosis for many of these couples.

• **Are the fallopian tubes open and normal?** The fallopian tubes provide the conduits for egg and sperm to meet. Conception occurs in the fallopian tube on the side of the body where the ovarian follicle releases the egg, and it is the job of the tubal fimbriae (fingerlike projections) to bring the egg into the tube. Inside the tubal lumen, or canal, fertilization takes place, along with early embryo development. A healthy fallopian tube has normal muscular contractions that will help the embryo migrate through the tubal canal to the uterus. Several medical problems can lead to permanent tubal blockage, including venereal diseases (gonorrhea and/or chlamydia), infection or scarring within the uterus, a ruptured appendix, or prior open abdominal surgical procedures, including cesarean section births.

A relatively easy test called a hysterosalpingogram (HSG) can usually determine if the fallopian tubes are open. The test is carried out in a radiology facility and requires the use of a small straw-like catheter at the entrance of the cervix. The test can cause some mild to moderate cramps but is usually well tolerated, especially if a cramp reliever like ibuprofen is taken one hour before the test. A small amount of clear contrast fluid is infused, and a fluoroscopic X-ray is taken to observe the progress of the fluid into the uterus and tubes. In thirty to sixty seconds it is usually possible to clearly witness X-ray fluid pouring out of the tubes. Blockages at any point within the tubes can be identified. An HSG test is not perfect and false positive readings can occur. Occasionally, the beginning muscular portions of the fallopian tubes will spasm, causing an artificial, temporary blockage.

Not all doctors perform an HSG on all Syndrome O women right from the outset. However, if there is anything about a patient's medical history that suggests fallopian tube disease, the test should be carried out *before* treatment cycles are initiated. This is an important judgment to make and requires informed discussion with all patients. Many women prefer to know that their fallopian tubes are definitely open before proceeding to fertility medication treatments. Even if the decision is made to initially defer the HSG, should two or three ovulation cycles prove unsuccessful, the HSG becomes even more important.

- **Are the fallopian tubes open, but possibly damaged?**
  Due to some false positive readings, an HSG can provide in-
  accurate reassurance that the fallopian tubes are normal. As I
  point out to my patients, the HSG only gives us some basic
  information about the internal plumbing of the tubes. However, the HSG can sometimes identify true abnormalities,
  such as a "clubbed" tube (significant damage and scarring of
  the fimbriae) or *hydrosalpinx* (stagnant fluid trapped in the
  tube). In these situations the tube(s) may be partially open but
  likely became severely damaged by prior infection or inflammation within the canal and muscular layers. Fallopian tubes
  that are affected by hydrosalpinx (or *hydrosalpinges* when both
  tubes are involved) may not only be nonfunctional, but may
  actually impede the ability of an embryo to implant within
  the uterus. There is a large body of literature demonstrating
  the negative effects of hydrosalpinges upon pregnancy rates
  following IVF treatment. Abnormal HSG findings might also
  mean that an outpatient surgical procedure called a *laparoscopy* (described below) will be recommended prior to any
  other fertility treatment.
- **Could pelvic adhesions or scar tissue block conception?**
  Fallopian tubes can appear normal on HSG, yet be wrapped
  in scar tissue or fixed in an abnormal spot within the pelvis.
  Prior infection, surgery, or endometriosis can contribute to this
  common problem, and a detailed medical history often suggests that further exploration is required. With a high index
  of suspicion, a laparoscopy should uncover such problems,
  which can often be corrected at the same procedure. Through
  three tiny openings in the skin, and under general anesthesia,
  an expert laparoscopy team can carefully evaluate both macro-
  and micro-adhesions, cut or remove excess scar tissue, free fallopian tubes from nonfunctional positions, check the fimbriae
  of the tubes, remove cysts (called paratubal cysts) hanging
  from the ends of the tubes, and generally restore normal
  anatomical relationships among the uterus, tubes, and ovaries.

In some instances it is appropriate to remove one or both damaged fallopian tubes via laparoscopy, since tubes that have become hydrosalpinges are unlikely to promote conception, and might actually interfere. A careful assessment by the laparoscopy team often provides vital information to help a couple evaluate their fertility care options. A recommendation of IVF is sometimes given, based on extensive and uncorrectable disease. Although this opinion may not initially be well received, it is foolhardy for a couple to waste time and money on non-IVF fertility cycles that are likely to be unsuccessful. Seeking second opinions can sometimes be reassuring, although the second doctor won't usually have had the benefit of visualizing the pelvis directly. The second doctor may have to base his or her opinions on the written report and pictures provided by the surgical team. Laparoscopy can be repeated (and sometimes really needs to be), but that puts additional burden, cost, and risk on the patient.

- **Are uterine polyps, fibroids, or hyperplastic changes present in the endometrium?** Polyps can occur in various parts of the body, but within the uterus they appear as tonguelike growths of tissue protruding into the inside cavity, or chamber, of the uterus. Uterine polyps usually consist primarily of endometrium, the glandular tissue that lines the inside of the uterus. As described in earlier chapters, the endometrium is quite responsive to pulses of estrogen, progesterone, and the insulin family of hormones. Syndrome O women are prone to exaggerated signals affecting the endometrium, including growth-inducing hormones that promote polyp formation. Most uterine polyps are benign when examined under the microscope, but they can interfere with embryo implantation and subsequent pregnancy development. Uterine fibroids (*myomas*) are relatively common benign muscle tumors resembling pearls and are not necessarily more common in women with Syndrome O. However, if fibroids grow into the uterine cavity, they will worsen the chances for achieving pregnancy, as well as increasing the possibility of miscarriage.

An abnormally thick endometrium measured by ultrasound warrants further investigation, particularly if no menses have occurred for many months. Of course, recent ovulation or early pregnancy must first be ruled out! It is worth repeating again that women who have ovarian confusion and ovulation disruption are at increased risk for precancerous (*hyperplastic*) changes, or even serious cancerous growth within the endometrium. Fortunately, three different complementary and important techniques exist for evaluating the endometrium closely.

As a first step, a specialized ultrasound, called a *sonohysterography*, provides a great deal of information about the anatomy of the endometrium. The sonohysterography (also

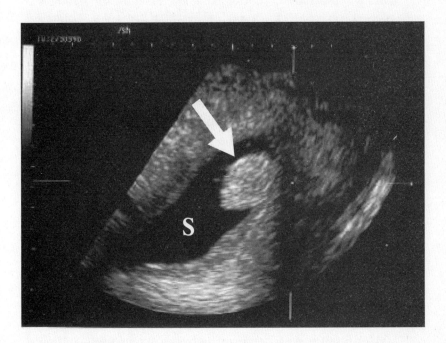

Sonohysterography (saline infusion ultrasound) demonstrating a prominent polyp (arrow) protruding into the uterine cavity. Dark fluid from the saline (S) provides excellent contrast and visualization of the flesh-toned polyp.

called *saline infusion sonography*) is performed by slowly instill-
ing a small amount of sterile saline liquid through the cervix
via a short plastic catheter. Simultaneously, a real-time ultrasound image of the fluid entering the uterus is seen. Most
women find this test very easy to undergo, because it causes
minimal or no cramps. They also find it quite fascinating as
they observe images of their uterus on the ultrasound screen.
Any abnormal structure protruding into the uterine cavity,
such as a polyp or fibroid, can be visualized and measured.
Interestingly, the X-ray HSG test has been shown to be much
less sensitive than the sonohysterography for evaluation of the
uterine cavity. Therefore, we commonly recommend both
tests as a full and complementary assessment of the uterus and
fallopian tubes.

If the uterine cavity appears clear of abnormalities by
sonohysterography, a thickened endometrium still requires
closer evaluation. This is done by "sampling," or removing a
small biopsy of the endometrium via a plastic device introduced into the uterus. It is common to experience about
twenty to thirty seconds of mild or moderate cramping during
the procedure. For sonohysterography or endometrial sampling, either ibuprofen or a similar cramp prevention medication is recommended one hour before test time. Ask your
doctor about pain medication before having the test done.

Many doctors believe that *hysteroscopy* is the gold standard
for best evaluating the endometrium, since this procedure allows an actual visualization of the inside of the uterus with a
camera. When performed in an outpatient surgery center,
general anesthesia can be administered, allowing the doctor to
dilate the cervix and comfortably place the hysteroscopic instrument within the uterus. This technique permits very clear
visualization of the uterine cavity, easy removal of polyps
and/or fibroids via accompanying hysteroscopic tools, and simultaneous and focused sampling of the endometrium. An
important benefit of hysteroscopy is that both diagnosis and

treatment can be carried out at the same procedure. Although some doctors perform hysteroscopy in their office, the procedure is often limited to "diagnosis only" in this setting. We prefer to utilize the sensitive sonohysterography test for initial diagnosis and proceed to therapeutic hysteroscopy only when warranted. However, if laparoscopy is already contemplated, we will commonly recommend hysteroscopy at that time.

- **Can the ovaries be seen clearly on transvaginal ultrasound?** In some cases, it can be very difficult to identify the position of the ovaries during transvaginal ultrasound. This problem seems more common in women with a markedly elevated BMI, particularly with individuals in the very obese range. When further evaluated by abdominal ultrasound, the ovaries are often identified in a higher abdominal position, often outside of the pelvis. Although laparoscopic evaluation sometimes demonstrates adhesions or cysts causing the ovaries to be abnormally located, the problem is more often caused by fatty tissue that has infiltrated the pelvis and tissues surrounding the small and large intestine. Extra stored fat can literally push the ovaries up and out of the pelvis because there is simply not enough room. Under normal circumstances, the ovaries and fallopian tubes should hang deep in the pelvis behind and on either side of the uterus. For some obese women this raises a significant concern that an egg released from an ovary might not easily be picked up by the fimbriae of the fallopian tube. Even during IVF procedures, ovaries located outside the pelvis provide a difficult and unsafe scenario for successful egg retrieval. Thus, in addition to the metabolic consequences of obesity, *anatomic distortion* of the reproductive organs because of fat distribution in the pelvis can impede fertility treatments.
- **Are thyroid and prolactin hormones normal?** The thyroid gland is a metabolic guard for the entire body, with every organ in the body requiring thyroid hormone action. Women are more prone than men to inflammation and autoimmune

attack upon the thyroid, and the implications on fertility and pregnancy can be profound. Recent recommendations urge that all reproductive age women be tested for normal thyroid function prior to and during pregnancy. If a pregnant woman's thyroid gland doesn't work properly, this can affect the neurological development of the fetus. A simple and sensitive blood test for thyroid stimulating hormone (TSH) can help diagnose early and more severe cases of *hypothyroidism* (underactive thyroid). For women who are trying to conceive, it appears prudent to treat mild hypothyroidism with monitored quantities of thyroid replacement medication. The TSH test can also point to *hyperthyroidism* (overactive thyroid), although this problem is much less common.

Irregular or absent menstrual cycles can sometimes be caused by an elevation in the hormone prolactin, secreted by the pituitary gland. Prolactin is an important hormone during and after pregnancy because of its role in stimulating breast milk production. However, if a small benign pituitary growth called an *adenoma* develops within the substance of the pituitary gland, excess prolactin from the adenoma will interfere with normal production of FSH and LH. Occasionally, a prolactin-producing adenoma will cause inappropriate breast milk production and secretion. Although prolactin adenomas are not specifically linked with Syndrome O, any woman with irregular or absent menses should be checked for elevated prolactin levels. An imaging test of the head, such as an MRI, is sensitive enough to diagnose a very tiny (as small as 1 to 2 mm) prolactin adenoma. Several medications are available to treat prolactin adenomas, with efficient restoration of ovulation and fertility.

- **How does age affect fertility?** It is likely that you were born with thousands of healthy eggs and follicles. Since birth, however, many eggs and follicles have withered away in a natural process called *atresia*. The process of atresia is not well understood, but heredity probably determines the rate of fol-

licular atresia and the actual age of menopause, a time when
the ovaries become completely depleted of eggs. Statistics
show that female fertility starts to gradually diminish at age
thirty, with sharper declines in the odds of conception seen
after age thirty-five and forty. The incidence of infertility increases dramatically as a function of age, and the effectiveness
of fertility treatments is very dependent on the age of the patient. Using the year 2000 U.S. IVF success rates as an indicator of age factors, thirty-year-old women had a 35 percent
success rate per IVF cycle attempt, whereas the birth rate
dropped considerably to 15 percent per cycle for forty-year-
old women, and 2 percent per cycle for forty-four-year-old
women. Public awareness campaigns have attempted to educate people about the impact of a woman's age upon fertility,
yet millions of couples delay seeking guidance and/or care
from specialists knowledgeable about this issue.

Age is also a major factor related to miscarriage risk, particularly during the first trimester of pregnancy. Older eggs
are more likely to harbor chromosome mistakes and other
abnormalities, rendering the resultant embryos and pregnancies nonviable. Most miscarriages are caused by an abnormal

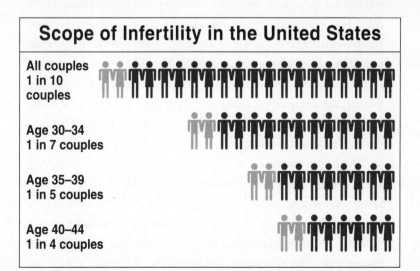

Scope of Infertility in the United States

All couples
1 in 10
couples

Age 30–34
1 in 7 couples

Age 35–39
1 in 5 couples

Age 40–44
1 in 4 couples

genetic makeup in the egg prior to conception and the risk of this problem increases dramatically with age. IVF statistics again underscore this fact. Once achieving a pregnancy with IVF, thirty-year-old women had an 11 percent risk of pregnancy loss, whereas the miscarriage rate at age forty was 29 percent, and at forty-four was 69 percent. The metabolic impact of Syndrome O heightens the risk of pregnancy loss at any age, and possible reasons for this are discussed in chapter 6.

- **Have preconception recommendations been provided?** In any given year in the United States, millions of couples are contemplating or actively working toward pregnancy and childbirth. When fertility issues such as Syndrome O get in the way of achieving a successful pregnancy, it is important to address a number of preconception issues *before* treatment begins. Although it is beyond the scope of this book to provide extensive details regarding preconception care, all readers (and their doctors) should be aware of a basic framework. Additional information can be obtained through official recommendations of the American College of Obstetricians and Gynecologists (www.acog.org). Another terrific source of factual information about fertility-related issues can be found on the Web site of the American Society for Reproductive Medicine (www.asrm.org). The March of Dimes (www.marchofdimes.com) has an excellent preconception screening and counseling checklist that can be downloaded in *pdf* format without cost. It is interesting to note that diet, exercise, and lifestyle receive top billing in the March of Dimes checklist. The following is a list of vital issues to consider:

  Medical problems that do not mix well with pregnancy. Preexisting health disorders or diseases involving the heart, lungs, liver, and kidneys may cause your pregnancy to be considered very high risk or possibly contraindicated. Certain vascular, autoimmune, neurologic, metabolic, genetic, and thrombotic disorders should be evaluated with regard to safety and possible treatment interventions during pregnancy. Details of prior surgery may also be important to review. Consultation and collaboration with relevant medical specialists and maternal fetal medicine (high-risk) doctors may be required and are best initiated *before* conception.

Medications that shouldn't be taken during pregnancy. The list is long, but your doctors should be made aware of every medicine you take currently or have taken in the recent past. Some medications are considered *teratogenic* (causing birth defects) and can linger in your body before it is safe to conceive. Although there is much interest and speculation around the world regarding the use of medicinal herbs for enhancing fertility, these cannot be endorsed at the current time. Some herbal preparations may seem harmless, but the long-ranging effects on the reproductive system, as well as the impact on embryonic and fetal development, are not known.

Infectious disease screens. It is considered prudent to test prospective parents for hepatitis, HIV, syphilis, and immunity to rubella (German measles) and varicella (chicken pox). If a concern is raised, tests for sexually transmitted diseases such as gonorrhea, chlamydia, herpes, and HPV (human papilloma virus) should be carried out. Cat owners may need testing for immunity to the parasite toxoplasmosis. A woman should have had a normal Pap smear within one year prior to conception.

Vaccinations. These are generally recommended one to three months prior to conception for women who are not immune to rubella and varicella. Women at higher risk for exposure to hepatitis B may also wish to consider immunization prior to conception.

Smoking and use of alcohol, caffeine, and recreational drugs. Here is a simple and terse recommendation—none of these are considered compatible with a safe and healthy pregnancy. High amounts of caffeine intake have been linked to miscarriage, so it is hard to know how lower amounts, even in a single daily cup of coffee, could affect a pregnancy.

Environmental factors. Numerous toxins and chemicals abound in our air, soil, and water, and these may impact fertility and pregnancy maintenance. While there is much finger pointing and uncertainty in this arena, it may be prudent to learn more about the air, water, and soil history in your workplace and at home. The U.S. Environmental Protection Agency (EPA) refers to certain toxins as "endocrine disrupters." These are chemicals that could interfere with normal glandular and reproductive processes in animals and humans. If you suspect there is a "cluster" of individuals with infertility and/or miscarriage occurring in your workplace, that may be an issue worth investigating with your employer and possibly even the U.S. Office of Occupational Health and Safety Administration (OSHA). OSHA (found at www.osha.gov) is responsible for overseeing the use of hazardous substances or toxins in the workplace. Both the EPA and the FDA have issued warnings about mercury and polychlorinated biphenyl (PCB) levels in our fresh fish food supply. Despite the overwhelming health benefits of fish and seafood, especially for Syndrome O women, some careful consideration of these advisories is warranted. Recently, even farm-raised fish were found to contain very high levels of PCBs.

Prenatal vitamins. Multivitamins, specifically those containing folic acid (400 µg/day), are strongly recommended. Folic acid prior to pregnancy promotes normal neural tube development in the fetus and helps prevent spina bifida and other neural tube defects. Untested and potentially harmful herbal and alternative medicine remedies should be avoided. You should let your doctor know about any supplements you're taking.

Genetic screening. Our growing knowledge about genes now permits laboratory testing for common inherited diseases, such as cystic fibrosis. The American College of Obstetricians and Gynecologists has recommended that carrier testing for cystic fibrosis be offered to all prospective parents. About 1 in 600 couples are at significant risk for having a child with cystic fibrosis. Despite ACOG's recommendation, many insurance carriers will not pay for this testing, which can cost $300 to $600. It is widely believed that genetic screening should also be offered for other severe diseases, such as fragile X (a common cause of mental retardation), sickle cell anemia (a blood disorder most common in people of African-American ancestry), thalasemia (a blood disorder common in people of Mediterranean and Far East ancestry), and Tay Sachs and Canavan's disease (most common in people of Ashkenazi Jewish heritage).

Genetic counseling and testing. Thousands of uncommon, yet severe and inherited diseases exist within families. Clinical geneticists and genetic counselors are experts in this rapidly growing area of medicine. They prefer to carry out their detective work regarding a rare genetic disease *before* conception, since that provides them with much needed time for research and possible testing of other family members. Huge worldwide computerized data banks regarding genetic diseases are updated daily and are readily available to these professionals. In many instances, prepregnancy embryo testing can be carried out in conjunction with IVF, a technique called pre-implantation genetic diagnosis (PGD). Thousands of couples are also counseled annually regarding age-related risks of having a baby with Down syndrome, caused by having a third #21 chromosome (or trisomy 21). Many other fetal chromosome abnormalities become more prevalent as the mother gets older. Experts in genetic counseling can help guide couples, usually once pregnant, as to what options are available for testing. Some couples may prefer a combination of noninvasive tests, such as fetal ultrasound and/or blood levels of certain hormones. Other couples may request more invasive tests, like amniocentesis (which checks fetal cells in amniotic fluid), or chorionic villus sampling (which tests the placenta cells from a first-trimester pregnancy). Genetic testing is a very personal choice and some couples prefer to avoid it altogether.

Picking a doctor and hospital. Hopefully you have already identified a women's health-care practitioner—in a solo or group practice—that meets your expectations for obstetrical and gynecological care. If so, consider yourself lucky in this regard, since many obstetrics and gynecology specialists around the country are closing their doors to new patients. Monumental changes in the insurance industry have put many doctors in a vice-like grip between lowered reimbursements for care and higher costs for malpractice liability, employee health coverage, and workman's compensation insurance. U.S. residency programs graduate about 1,100 newly minted specialists in obstetrics and gynecology each year, with most becoming board-certified within two to five years. However, many of these specialists choose nonobstetrical subspecialties (oncology, pelvic surgery, urology, and reproductive endocrinology) or opt for research careers in academic institutions and pharmaceutical companies. Some even work as writers! Referrals to state-of-the-art obstetrical practices commonly come from primary-care doctors, fertility specialists, local hospitals, or by word of mouth. Hospitals that provide obstetrical services should also have opportunities for educational sessions, prenatal classes, and rapid access to specialized nursery care. Your pregnancy outcome can be dramatically affected by the availability of sophisticated maternal, fetal, and neonatal medicine care in your community.

A Plan of Attack

A diligent investigation of all fertility and Syndrome O factors, along with a thorough assessment of preconception issues, can usually be completed in two to four weeks following initial consultation. If a hysteroscopy and/or laparoscopy are recommended, additional time might be required to accommodate procedure scheduling and post-operative recuperation. You might find it helpful to maintain an ongoing personal calendar of tests as they are recommended and completed, since it will serve as a useful framework for future discussions with your doctor.

- **What is wrong with me (us)?** Before initiating any treatment regimen, a detailed follow-up consultation with your doctor should focus on: 1) your test results and those of your partner; 2) conclusions regarding female and/or male fertility factors; and 3) a logical plan of attack. Based on your doctor's judgment and interpretation of your test results, an accurate diagnostic list should then be formulated. For many women with Syndrome O it is common to find no other interfering fertility factors, and this conclusion should be viewed as good news. However, results pointing to a severe male factor and/or certain female fertility problems detailed above might necessitate more advanced fertility care, such as IVF.

  A diagnosis of Syndrome O or polycystic ovaries should prompt some personal reflection and goal setting before immediately moving ahead with fertility treatments. With your whole body affected in different ways by overnourishment and insulin overproduction, it is logical to assume that your ovaries and reproductive system will be less apt to respond effectively to fertility medications. Organized and optimized life changes in your nutrition, activity, stress, and relationships with yourself and others—the Syndrome O Survival

(SOS) Strategies—will maximize treatment effectiveness while minimizing time and costs. Chapter 9 is entirely devoted to a detailed description of the SOS Strategies.

- **What are our chances of getting pregnant?** It would thrill me to tell every couple seeking fertility care that they have a 100 percent chance of achieving pregnancy. We all know this would be overly optimistic and untruthful. However, before a couple makes a significant investment of time, emotions, and dollars, it is advantageous to provide an educated estimate of success. Important factors like age, severity of disease, prior fertility, and outcome of prior treatments can either impede or enhance the prognosis.

Fecundity is the scientific term given to describe the likelihood of conception in a female ovulatory cycle. Most people are surprised to learn that even in the best of circumstances— a younger, fertile, ovulating, sperm-producing, motivated couple having sexual relations on a regular basis—there is only a 20 percent chance of conceiving each month. After six months of trying, that same couple has a cumulative chance of conception approaching 75 to 80 percent. For a forty-year-old woman with no other infertility factors, the estimated chance of conception is about 5 percent each month.

Normal fecundity is reduced by numerous factors, including Syndrome O. When a woman does not ovulate, fecundity essentially drops to zero. Factors such as blocked fallopian tubes, pelvic adhesions, and severe male infertility will also cause a fecundity rate of zero. Advancing age will gradually reduce fecundity, with significant decreases noted after ages thirty-five and forty. Fertility treatments become less effective with advancing age.

The goal of conservative fertility treatment is to improve fecundity to a level compatible with natural conception rates for other women the same age. *Ovulation induction* is the clinical term used to describe treatments for overcoming ovulation disruption and ovarian confusion associated with Syndrome

O. Under optimal circumstances—when effective insulin-lowering strategies have been implemented—ovulation should be relatively easy to induce. When strategically inclined Syndrome O women undergo ovulation induction, their chances of getting pregnant are similar to other women their age who ovulate regularly and spontaneously. For most women under thirty, this translates into a 20 percent chance of conception with each monthly cycle of ovulation induction, assuming no other barriers to conception have been found. Between ages thirty and forty, most women with Syndrome O under control should have an age-appropriate chance of conception of 10 to 20 percent during each ovulatory cycle. Although IVF often provides better odds of conception per treatment cycle, the costs are high. Ovulation induction is still the most prudent and cost-effective first-line therapy for helping Syndrome O women achieve pregnancy.

- **Will treatments be painful?** Aside from the distaste many women have regarding blood tests, ultrasound, and pelvic examination, it is safe to say that most treatments involving ovulation induction are not painful.

- **Will I have a multiple pregnancy?** This is a vital area of concern for many patients, their doctors, and the health insurance industry. Although twins occur naturally in about 1 to 2 percent of pregnancies, higher order multiples (triplets, quadruplets, etc.) are much rarer. Statistics kept by the Centers for Disease Control indicate that since 1980, fertility care services have been solely responsible for the dramatic increase in twins and high-order multiples. About half of these pregnancies have occurred with IVF and the rest are related to ovulation induction. Many are attributable to poorly monitored and/or overly aggressive ovulation induction cycles and excessive numbers of embryos transferred to the uterus at one time. Informed consent for any fertility treatment necessitates a frank discussion of this issue. Overly aggressive ovulation induction cycles with gonadotropins should be a thing of the past for most patients. Intelligent IVF care generally limits embryo transfer numbers to two. If carried out properly, less than 10 percent of successful ovulation induction cycles should result in twins, and less than 1 percent should yield triplets. The twin pregnancy rate with IVF remains high in many clinics (25 to 40 percent of pregnancies), but triplet rates are progressively dropping to below 5 percent of all IVF pregnancies. In the year 2000, 31 percent of IVF live births in the United States were twins, and 4 percent were triplets. With the increasing utilization of single embryo transfers, multiple pregnancy rates from IVF should steadily decline.

• **How much will all this cost?** Although many of the best things in life are free, fertility care rarely qualifies. In order to provide top-notch service, strict attention to detail, and round-the-clock expertise, your team of doctors, nurses, embryologists, and other staff are a well-integrated but expensive enterprise. Unlike other aspects of medical care, insurance coverage for fertility treatments can vary dramatically from state to state, and from employer to employer. Most reputable fertility clinics will provide written details of costs and insurance benefits before starting treatment. Many clinics provide options for financing. Two of the largest companies in the United States to offer fertility care financing are Advanced Reproductive Care (www.arcfertility.com) and IntegraMed (www.integramed.com). Each of these companies comprises a large network of participating fertility specialists around the country. Like housing prices, the cost of fertility care can vary by geographic region, population density, and clinics present in a certain locale. There are currently about 425 IVF clinics in the United States performing more than 100,000 cycles per year, supervised by about 800 board-certified and/or board-eligible reproductive endocrinologists in active clinical practice. In the near future, the number of infertile couples seeking care—about 1 million per year—

will dramatically outpace the number of trained specialists able to provide that care. This is an important issue for Syndrome O women to consider as they explore and develop personal life-enhancing strategies to maximize their treatment success. For many couples, cost issues weigh heavily on their decision making. I have witnessed (and even encouraged) some couples changing jobs or moving to states that mandate infertility insurance coverage.

- **What if treatments are not successful?** There is no easy answer to this dilemma. With appropriate guidance from doctors, nurses, and counselors, it is sometimes appropriate to stop treatment and consider other family-building options. Nonprofit national consumer advocacy organizations like RESOLVE (www.resolve.org) and the American Infertility Association (www.americaninfertility.org) provide information, seminars, and other resources for couples interested in adoption. Many other couples pursue alternatives like donor egg, donor sperm, uterine surrogacy, and embryo adoption. The more questions you ask, the more answers you will find. Always consider second, or even third opinions before making final decisions. Persistence in finding honest answers and guidance often can be fruitful, even when the prognosis seems bleak.

CLOMIPHENE: A FERTILITY DRUG TO BE THANKFUL FOR

Drug discovery often takes unexpected turns, as evidenced by the observation in the 1950s that clomiphene induces ovulation. With rising incidences of breast and endometrial cancer during the mid-twentieth century, scientists were eager to develop medications to counteract tumor growth stimulated by estrogen. Two structurally related anti-estrogen compounds first synthesized in the 1950s—clomiphene and tamoxifen—offered some hope for these estrogen-dependent cancers. Tamoxifen (Nolvadex) is now widely used for breast cancer treatment, whereas clomiphene (Clomid, Serophene) is the primary oral medication prescribed for ovulation induction. Since the first published description of clomiphene use for ovulation induction in 1961 by Dr. R. B. Greenblatt, millions of babies have been conceived.

Clomiphene induces follicular growth by a two-step process. First, as an anti-estrogen, it tricks the hypothalamus and the pituitary gland into producing enhanced amounts of follicle stimulating hormone (FSH). This boost of FSH in the bloodstream then signals growth and

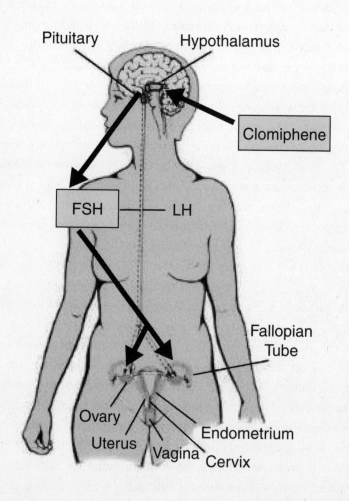

Potential Adverse Reactions to Clomiphene

Ovarian enlargement:

- Residual cysts or unruptured follicles
- Ruptured cyst with bleeding
- Ovarian torsion (twisting)
- Abdominal bloating or distention

Ovarian hyperstimulation syndrome:

- Abdominal bloating, distention, and pain
- Nausea and/or vomiting
- Weight gain
- Dehydration and/or poor urine production

Visual symptoms:

- Blurred or double vision
- Flashing lights, floaters, "waves"
- Photophobia (aversion to light)
- Dizziness

Headache

Mood changes:

- Worsening depression
- Irritability and mood swings
- Anxiousness

Breast tenderness

If you are taking clomiphene and experience any of these symptoms, consult with your doctor.

development of granulosa cells within the follicle. In an uncontrolled Syndrome O environment of excess insulin and androgens, the additional FSH may not be effective and follicles will often not grow. Clomiphene works best if insulin and androgen levels have been normalized prior to and during treatment.

For women with Syndrome O, clomiphene is the mainstay of conservative therapy for ovulation induction. Even with worsening trends in insulin overproduction over the past twenty-five years, most Syndrome O women will ovulate when treated with an appropriate dose of clomiphene. Since clomiphene is considered safe, many gynecologists will prescribe it. Because there can be a wide disparity in response among patients, I have prescribed dosages as small as 25 mg for three days, or as high as 200 mg for ten days.

In many instances, ovarian response to the drug is not monitored closely by the prescribing physician, and other metabolic and fertility factors have not been considered. Therefore, most reproductive endocrinologists (including myself) do not endorse an unmonitored approach, since it often wastes valuable time and places women at higher risk for large ovarian cysts and multiple gestations. The box on page 91 lists potential adverse reactions to clomiphene, which fortunately occur in less than 2 percent of carefully monitored patients.

Each treatment attempt with clomiphene should be approached thoughtfully and thoroughly. Prior to taking clomiphene, a baseline ultrasound is strongly recommended to rule out large ovarian cysts and to evaluate the endometrial lining. It is also recommended that normal menses should have occurred, either induced by progesterone or by birth control pills. The clomiphene dosage prescribed may depend on prior response. For women who have never taken clomiphene, a common starting regimen is one 50-mg pill a day starting on cycle day five and continuing for five consecutive days. The first day of menstrual bleeding is considered cycle day one.

With strategic life changes instituted prior to treatment and maintained consistently, doctors can expect a 75 to 80 percent positive ovulatory response with a clomiphene regimen of 50 mg for five days.

Ultrasound monitoring starting several days after the last clomiphene pill is a wise policy. In some instances, follicular response can be robust, placing some women at risk for multiple egg release. The overall rate of twin conceptions is cited as 7 percent of clomiphene-induced pregnancies, but occasional conceptions of triplets (0.5 percent), quadruplets (0.3 percent), or quintuplets (0.1 percent) can occur. As part of informed consent, all couples should be counseled about this risk prior to treatment. If ultrasound monitoring demonstrates two or more developing follicles during a treatment cycle, the chance of multiple pregnancy is higher, and your clinical care team should discuss this with you.

If no follicular growth can be documented by ultrasound up to two weeks after the last pill was taken, you might be resistant to clomiphene. The reasons for this can be an insufficient release of FSH from the pituitary gland and/or a lack of follicular response to the FSH that was produced. From a practical standpoint it is impossible to distinguish these two mechanisms, but many women can benefit from increasing the dose and/or number of days of treatment. As the amount of clomiphene is increased in subsequent cycles, ultrasound monitoring becomes even more important. In addition, higher dosages of clomiphene can exert some significant *anti-estrogen effects* on endometrial growth and cervical mucus production, particularly if prescribed for three or more consecutive months.

True clomiphene resistance is found in 10 to 20 percent of Syndrome O women, and may be variably defined by different clinicians. Traditionally, the recommended *total* clomiphene dosage, according to the *2003 Physicians' Desk Reference,* should not exceed 500 mg in one month. With the increasing use of insulin-sensitizing medications as adjuncts to clomiphene ovulation induction, it may be wise to reevaluate the situation if clomiphene alone fails to stimulate follicular growth at that threshold. A lack of ovulation or response to clomiphene can also be seen in some women who do *not* have Syndrome O or polycystic ovaries. Prompt scrutiny of the original diagnosis is recommended.

When well-monitored attempts at ovulation induction fail to achieve follicular growth, alternate clomiphene-based regimens can be considered. Different clinicians may have certain rationales for the approach they recommend and it is important for you to be given that information in advance. Make sure you ask your doctor to explain his or her rationale for treatment.

- **Clomiphene with insulin sensitizers.** Insulin sensitizers are oral medications approved by the Food and Drug Administration for the treatment of type 2 diabetes. They function by allowing insulin to work more efficiently in the muscles, liver, and other organs. Two important jobs of these medications are to control blood sugar levels and to ease insulin overproduction and stress on the pancreas. Although not approved by the FDA for nondiabetic individuals, many clinicians and researchers believe that insulin sensitizers can help prevent the onset of diabetes. Furthermore, since insulin overproduction is central to Syndrome O fertility problems, insulin sensitizers can help ease ovarian confusion and ovulation disruption. In 1996, Dr. John Nestler first reported the impact of metformin (Glucophage) upon ovarian function, follicle growth, and ovulation. Since that time, metformin and two other insulin sensitizers—pioglitazone (Actos) and rosiglitazone (Avandia)—have been widely prescribed to Syndrome O women. Several peer-reviewed articles and numerous presentations at national meetings have demonstrated the benefit of insulin sensitizers as adjuncts for clomiphene-induced ovulation. Many women who are initially clomiphene-resistant will eventually ovulate if treated in conjunction with clomiphene and an insulin sensitizer. Additional prospective clinical trials are needed and at the time of this writing such studies are in progress through the National Institutes of Health and the national Reproductive Medicine Unit. More detailed information regarding the potential usefulness of insulin sensitizers will be provided in chapter 8.

- **Clomiphene followed by low-dose gonadotropins.** When clomiphene, with or without insulin sensitizers, doesn't induce follicle growth it may mean that additional help from FSH and LH hormones is required. As will be described in greater detail in the next chapter, injectable gonadotropins can provide direct FSH stimulation of the ovaries. Certain protocols for ovulation induction combine clomiphene and gonadotropins, typically in a sequential fashion. As an example, a patient may take clomiphene for five to seven days, followed by daily injections of low dose FSH (brand names Bravelle, Gonal-F, or Follistim). The rationale for this approach is that clomiphene gets things started by instructing the pituitary gland to release extra FSH and LH. Daily injections of FSH hopefully keep the momentum going by promoting gradual follicle growth. Close monitoring by ultrasound and blood hormone levels of estradiol are strongly advised. The responsiveness of the reproductive system to gonadotropin injections is often different for Syndrome O women, and the risks of pregnancy complications are higher. Multiple gestations heighten these risks substantially.

- **Clomiphene with dexamethasone.** Some clinicians advocate suppression of adrenal androgens with dexamethasone as a modality for helping ovarian function, follicle growth, and ovulation. Except for specific instances of an uncommon inherited problem called adrenal hyperplasia, this approach does not have widespread support. Cortisol-like drugs such as dexamethasone and prednisone clearly worsen insulin overproduction, and should be avoided except for specific medical indications.

- **Tamoxifen and aromatase inhibitors.** Some clinicians prefer prescribing tamoxifen (Nolvadex) as an alternative to clomiphene for ovulation induction. Tamoxifen is a cousin drug to clomiphene, but it is utilized and FDA approved primarily as an adjunctive treatment for breast cancer. When taken for five days, its mechanism of action in promoting pituitary FSH and LH release is similar to clomiphene. For the relatively small number of women who experience side effects from clomiphene (see the box on page 91), tamoxifen may be preferable. Although it has been proposed that tamoxifen may also be worth trying for anovulatory women who are clomiphene resistant, a recent prospective study demonstrated that overall rates of ovulation and pregnancy are similar between the two drugs. A newer class of oral breast cancer drugs, aromatase inhibitors, have also been prescribed in short daily bursts to women with Syndrome O. These drugs promote pituitary release of FSH and LH. Preliminary published studies by Dr. R. F. Casper and colleagues in Toronto, Canada, have demonstrated encouraging results with the aromatase inhibitor letrozole (Femara), even in women who have been resistant to clomiphene. Some clinicians believe that aromatase inhibitors may eventually replace clomiphene as the preferred method of conservative ovulation induction. Additional studies to better define the pros and cons of drugs like letrozole are currently underway.

The Big O: Ovulation

Induction of single follicle growth by conservative, cost-effective, and well-monitored treatments is the major goal of modern fertility care for Syndrome O women. However, follicle growth does not guarantee that ovulation will actually take place. As described in chapter 2, final maturation of the egg and enzymatic breakdown of the follicle wall require *luteinizing hormone* (LH). Many women are familiar with the concept of the LH surge, which is the normal outpouring of LH from the pituitary gland into the bloodstream twenty-four to thirty-six hours prior to ovulation.

Scientists understand a great deal about the glandular internet communication that takes place in the hypothalamus, pituitary, and ovarian follicle just before ovulation. Many Syndrome O women will not have an adequate surge of LH prior to ovulation or an effective response to LH within the follicle. It is also possible that insulin over-production may disrupt the delicate balance of enzymes in the follicle, which help break the follicle wall and permit extrusion of the egg at the proper time.

Scientists have been working on purifying medications that will help release the egg at the proper time. As of this writing, genetically engineered LH medication is available in Europe (Luveris) and other countries around the world, but not in the United States (pending FDA approval). As a medication, LH may have value during the different phases of ovulation induction treatments. Currently, an LH analog called *human chorionic gonadotropin* (HCG) is commonly used when the LH surge is absent or suboptimal. Many reproductive endocrinologists utilize a single well-timed HCG injection, administered either subcutaneously (Ovidrel) or intramuscularly (Novarel, Pregnyl, Profasi). In many fertility centers this is a routine approach for helping to ensure follicular wall breakdown and egg release. Other benefits to the use of HCG may include enhanced and prolonged stimulation of the corpus luteum, the progesterone-producing unit of the follicle.

Following a well-monitored ovulation induction cycle and administration of HCG, it may be appropriate to recommend an intrauterine insemination (IUI) procedure. Fertility specialists commonly recommend IUI in the setting of mild to moderate male factor infertility, or if cervical factors are suspected. As an anti–estrogen, clomiphene can interfere with normal cervical mucus production, creating a potentially hostile barrier for sperm penetration. Intrauterine inseminations are rarely painful and usually require only a few minutes. Preparation of the sperm in the laboratory for IUI requires sixty to ninety minutes. An IUI can be carried out once or twice during the thirty-six-hour time interval after HCG administration. Each case should be individualized, and the additional cost for the sperm preparation and IUI procedures should be disclosed prior to treat-

ment. Whether or not IUI is carried out, intercourse is highly recommended as spontaneously as possible three to five times during the
week prior to ovulation.

Doctors often prescribe progesterone following ovulation and inseminations. If the endometrial lining of the uterus was stimulated
properly with estrogen while follicle(s) were growing, it is likely that
the endometrium can secrete key substances after ovulation to enhance embryo implantation. Progesterone supplementation can aid
this process. Although natural progesterone can be taken orally or
administered by intramuscular injection, many clinicians prefer the
vaginal route, either with suppositories or gel (Crinone, Prochieve).
Research with vaginal progesterone has shown that there is faster accumulation in the uterus, as compared with oral or intramuscular administration. If pregnancy occurs, progesterone supplementation is
usually continued until the eleventh or twelfth week. In addition to
promoting the secretion of important endometrial substances, progesterone may also serve to relax the uterine musculature and enhance blood flow to the early developing conception.

If ovulation induction with clomiphene has not been successful
for you, do not despair. In many instances, uncontrolled Syndrome O
has interfered with clomiphene's effectiveness. Alternatively, there
may be male or other female factors that could necessitate more advanced treatments. Continue to ask questions and to seek logical answers. Help your doctors help you by being truthful and open to
ideas. Let no barriers be insurmountable in your quest to build your
family.

THE MOON CAN RISE—KEY POINTS TO KEEP IN MIND

Millions of women with Syndrome O, as well as other fertility problems, must consider their treatment options carefully. The good
news is that success is within your grasp. Some key points from this
chapter are:

- The number of couples suffering with infertility in the United States—estimated to be 5 million—is staggering, with Syndrome O contributing to 25 to 30 percent of female-factor cases.

- The availability of good fertility care information through books and the Internet can be helpful, yet overwhelming for many people. There is no substitution for a diligent and thorough evaluation by a trained fertility specialist prior to treatment.

- Syndrome O is diagnosed through a detailed medical history, physical examination, ultrasound, and specific blood studies. Related medical problems such as diabetes, glucose intolerance, hypertension, and androgen excess can be diagnosed and should be properly treated prior to conception. Treatment for Syndrome O involves a partnership with your doctor and a realistic effort to make personal life-management changes.

- Other fertility factors, both male and female, must be ruled out before proceeding to treatment. Basic evaluation of the sperm count and potential female pelvic factors must be considered. Patent fallopian tubes by HSG do not always indicate normally functioning tubes.

- Age is a significant factor when considering chances for success with any fertility treatment. Statistics from IVF are helpful to stress the impact of age on conception rates and miscarriage risk.

- Clomiphene is the mainstay of therapy for ovulation induction. Its value as a medication for inducing ovulation was discovered by chance in the 1950s. Many different protocols exist for clomiphene administration, but clomiphene resistance is a significant concern for many Syndrome O women.

- The positive effects of insulin sensitizers upon ovarian function underscore the impact of overnourishment and insulin overproduction in Syndrome O–related infertility. Specific life management strategies to lower insulin production and enhance fertility may be just as effective as insulin sensitizer drugs.

- The LH surge is required to induce enzymes in the follicle for expulsion of the mature egg. Ovulation can be augmented by administering HCG at the proper time. Intrauterine inseminations and luteal-phase progesterone support may help promote conception.

- Advanced and higher-tech fertility care may be necessary for more complex infertility cases. Coping with this possibility may become challenging to you on several levels—emotionally, financially, and physically. Educating yourself with the information you need to deal with fertility care issues can be very empowering. Don't despair. Expert professionals and support systems are out there to help you achieve success with your family-building endeavors.

- Fertility care patients approach their need for treatment in many different ways. It is hard to generalize and folly to assume that most people are having major emotional problems dealing with infertility. While going through treatments, most couples are actually upbeat and optimistic. Most women with Syndrome O are ultimately successful, even though family-building options may come in different packages.

FIVE

WHEN MORE ADVANCED FERTILITY CARE BECOMES NECESSARY

AN INJECTABLE KICK

Many different scientific and medical breakthroughs have converged over the past century to provide fertility specialists and their patients with tremendous options for safe and rational care. Advanced fertility care must be offered with a sound ethical foundation, and couples should be provided with thorough information regarding treatment benefits and potential risks. This is commonly referred to as *informed consent.* One unique feature of the fertility specialty is that joint decisions made by prospective parents and their doctors can have profound implications for the health and well-being of children long after they are born.

Syndrome O adds a special perspective to this process, but also an opportunity for women and their doctors. The Syndrome O phenomenon provides a wake-up call for women regarding their future health and life. The utilization of advanced fertility care—treatments such as ovulation induction with gonadotropins and *in vitro* fertilization (IVF)—has special considerations for women with Syndrome O.

For example, their sensitivity to insulin and gonadotropin hormones can add extra risk during fertility treatments. Once pregnant, miscarriage and high-risk pregnancies are more common among women with Syndrome O (discussed in chapters 6 and 7). Multiple gestation heightens risks substantially for all women. The purpose of this chapter is to review options for advanced fertility care and to provide general guidelines for women working to outsmart Syndrome O. But remember, no book or Web site information is intended or capable of being a substitute for individualized evaluation and treatment in the hands of expert physicians.

Early in the twentieth century, medical scientists concluded that the pituitary gland, embedded deep in the head near the brain, is a master gland influencing body growth, metabolism, and puberty, including the female menstrual cycle. By the 1930s, it was established that the pituitary gland produced one or more substance(s)—*gonadotrophic* hormones—that coursed through the blood stream to the *gonads,* affecting their growth and function: ovaries in women; testes in men.

Fascinating scientific discoveries about pituitary hormones have led to the development of gonadotropin medications, which continue to help millions of people around the world. Although early experiments showed that pituitary gland extracts could stimulate ovarian growth and follicle development, scientists debated whether one or two hormones were involved. In female monkeys, which have menstrual cycles similar to humans, pituitary extract induced follicles to grow. One active pituitary hormone was later called *follicle stimulating hormone* (FSH). However, a second pituitary hormone, now known as *luteinizing hormone* (LH), was also required to bring about follicle rupture and release of the egg (ovulation).

Scientists and doctors knew that it would never be practical to prepare pituitary extract as a medication for millions of people. But in the 1920s, pioneer researchers Drs. Ascheim and Zondek found that the urine of menopausal women contained hormones with potent activity identical to pituitary gonadotropins. This remarkable discovery was made because women's pituitary glands produce very high amounts of FSH and LH after menopause, as the growth of their

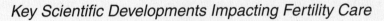

Key Scientific Developments Impacting Fertility Care

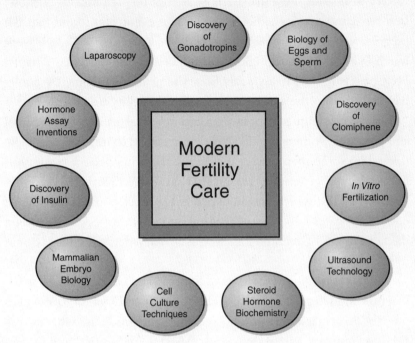

ovarian follicles and eggs wane. Menopausal women have very high amounts of FSH and LH in their bloodstream and urine, compared to reproductive age and pre-adolescent females.

The Serono company was the first to develop a urinary human menopausal gonadotropin (hMG) injectable medication—Pergonal—for use by infertile couples. This was a major medical and technologic breakthrough, particularly because the production of hMG required the collection and processing of millions of gallons of urine. From a particularly poignant viewpoint, menopausal women (including thousands of nuns in Europe) have donated their urine for decades to help millions of young couples throughout the world achieve their dreams.

The two active hormones in Pergonal—FSH and LH—work very efficiently to induce follicular growth. However, more scientific discoveries were needed for doctors to best understand how to mimic the important midcycle LH surge required for actual ovulation. For a variety of reasons, Pergonal alone could not be used for this purpose. In a separate series of experiments, it was eventually found that the pregnancy hormone *human chorionic gonadotropin* (HCG) acts very much like LH, even though it is produced by the placenta. Purified HCG, prepared for many years from the urine of pregnant women, has been vital to the success of virtually all fertility treatments.

Gonadotropin medications prepared from the urine of menopausal and pregnant women are still actively prescribed to millions of people (including some men). Since the 1990s, there has been a steady shift to the use of genetically engineered (also called *recombinant*) FSH, LH, and HCG, which are produced by genetically modified cells in culture. Debates continue in medical and scientific circles regarding the advantages of recombinant versus urinary-derived gonadotropin medicines.

Three companies in the United States have FDA approval to manufacture and sell gonadotropins. The Serono and Organon companies offer both urinary-derived and recombinant products, whereas the Ferring company sells just urinary-derived medications. Despite spirited and competitive marketing often put forth by these companies, it remains an open scientific question as to whether one particular gonadotropin product is superior to another. Educated consumers and insurance companies often take pricing considerations into account, since a single vial of gonadotropins may range widely in price from about $35 to $70 retail in the United States.

The role of LH prior to ovulation and egg release has been an area of active interest in scientific and pharmaceutical circles. Women with Syndrome O often produce extra LH, relative to FSH, and tend to have ovaries that produce higher amounts of androgens as a result. As discussed previously, insulin overproduction worsens the situation. Therefore, many doctors will try to tailor ratios of FSH and LH when they decide which gonadotropin medications to prescribe. In many instances, follicle growth can be induced with FSH alone in women with Syndrome O, followed by actual ovulation brought about by a single injection of HCG.

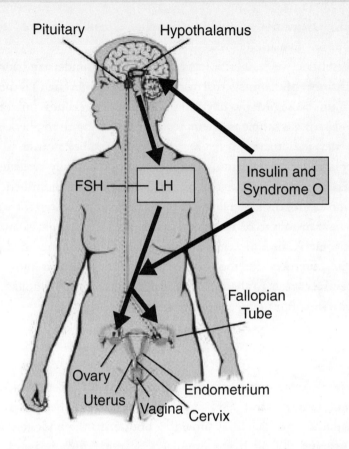

MONITORING THE SITUATION

Many women come to my office stating "I took clomiphene but it didn't work." From their perspective, "not working" usually equates with not becoming pregnant. Often, these women were prescribed clomiphene by their gynecologist but the effect of the clomiphene wasn't monitored by ultrasound or blood hormone levels. Occasionally, incomplete monitoring was performed and included tests such as a single ultrasound to assess follicle growth and/or a single progesterone level. In general, unsuccessful results with clomiphene fall into three common categories: 1) clomiphene did induce follicle growth, but a lack of LH surge failed to bring about follicle rupture and egg release; 2) clomiphene induced follicle growth and ovulation, but no pregnancy occurred; and 3) clomiphene neither induced follicle growth nor ovulation.

Reproductive endocrinologists are trained to understand and treat disturbances of the menstrual cycle, of which Syndrome O is the most common cause. Many physicians in other specialties misconstrue anovulation as a simple problem, readily treatable by clomiphene alone. However, the situation is rarely that simple. Metabolic causes of ovarian confusion and ovulation disruption must be carefully evaluated and treated before prescribing any medication for ovulation induction.

Gonadotropins may be the most appropriate next step for women who have proven to be resistant to clomiphene. However, as discussed in chapter 4, insulin sensitizers may help clomiphene work, thus avoiding the need for more expensive, riskier gonadotropins. There are several caveats to the use of gonadotropins, which should fall under the important concept of informed consent.

The Purpose of Gonadotropins

As injectable medicines, gonadotropins can provide specific quantities of biologically active FSH and LH directly into the bloodstream. Generally, these injections provide a booster to the endogenous gonadotropins already being produced by the pituitary gland. Since some Syndrome O women are often producing mild or moderately increased quantities of endogenous LH, most fertility experts favor purified FSH for ovulation induction, rather than hMG (which contains FSH and LH). Purified FSH is sold as genetically engineered Gonal-F (Serono) or Follistim (Organon), or as urinary-derived Bravelle (Ferring).

Even in a setting of clomiphene resistance, FSH should be prescribed gingerly, since the initial response may be unpredictable. The goal to be achieved is the growth induction of one dominant follicle. Many practitioners, including myself, will initiate treatment with 37.5 to 75 units (one-half to one full vial or ampule) of FSH on the third day of the menstrual period, with a gradual "step-up" in dosing by 37.5 to 75 units if needed. It is crucial for doctors to determine the rate of follicle growth, as well as the number of follicles that are growing. This is done by transvaginal ultrasound, sometimes daily. Along with ultrasound monitoring, most fertility specialists will check the accompanying levels of estradiol, progesterone, and LH in the blood. This information helps determine the progress and safety of the cycle and allows for proper medication decisions.

In order to minimize the risk of multiple gestation, it is wise for couples to avoid intercourse until the cycle's progress clearly yields a desired conservative response—one or possibly two growing follicles. Final egg maturity, as well as ovulation, is commonly achieved after a single injection of HCG, at the discretion of the practitioner monitoring the cycle.

Conservative use of gonadotropins by this step-up approach helps promote single follicle growth and successful pregnancies. For many couples, patience is a virtue. However, for many women with Syndrome O, this path to ovulation may require twenty-one to twenty-eight days, or longer, creating weariness and frustration. It helps significantly to explain the individualized nature and clear-cut advantages of this approach in advance of the treatment cycle.

Pituitary and Ovarian Suppression

Many fertility specialists believe that reducing ovarian androgens prior to and during a treatment cycle can be beneficial in promoting healthy follicular growth. One good option for reducing androgens is the short-term use of birth control pills (BCP), overlapped with the use of a gonadotropin-suppressing drug such as leuprolide (Lupron). In this setting, the BCP is part of the treatment; it is not being used to prevent pregnancy! Typically, the BCP is taken for a minimum of three weeks, with a one-week overlap of daily subcutaneous leuprolide. The BCP is then stopped, but the leuprolide is continued. Once a menstrual period occurs, gonadotropin induction can start at any point. Leuprolide dosing is often reduced once gonadotropins are started.

Although this approach adds time and expense to the cycle, reliable reductions in pituitary LH and ovarian androgens are seen, thus improving the ovarian environment. In this setting, higher initial doses of gonadotropins may be required and conservative combinations of FSH and hMG are often utilized to provide both FSH and LH. Leuprolide gonadotropin suppression has been the mainstay of ovulation induction for *in vitro* fertilization for many years and does not appear harmful to egg or embryo development.

Controlling Insulin Overproduction Before Ovulation Therapy

Insulin, along with insulinlike hormones (like IGF-I), act as cogonadotropins. The impact of the insulin hormone family can be quite important to cells within the ovaries that may receive improper hormone instructions to overproduce androgens. Although some in-

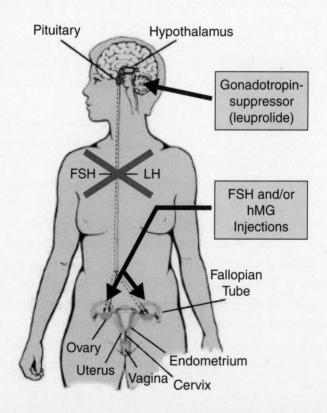

sulin and androgens are absolutely necessary for healthy follicle and egg development, Syndrome O dramatically confuses the ovarian environment. Ovulation induction with gonadotropins can be inefficient and sometimes downright dangerous in a setting of uncontrolled insulin overproduction.

Even if the pituitary gland and ovaries are suppressed with BCP or leuprolide, insulin continues to provide a stimulus for ovarian androgen production. It seems prudent to initiate and maintain a personal plan for reducing overnourishment and insulin overproduction before and during any fertility treatment.

However, many fertility specialists are quite skeptical of their patients' ability to maintain an insulin-lowering plan and would rather prescribe insulin-lowering medications, such as glucophage, pioglitazone, or rosiglitazone. Such doctors claim it is easier to just prescribe medications, rather than offering some honest discussions and counseling about obesity, insulin resistance, and healthy alternatives to overnourishment. Physician partnerships with nonprofit groups such as PCOStrategies (www.pcostrategies.org) can often provide the necessary education, motivation, and proactive stimulation for Syndrome O women desiring fertility and good health without medications.

On the flip side, other practitioners downright refuse to offer fertility treatments to women who are above a certain BMI, especially if other medical problems exist. The argument offered by these doctors is that pregnancy is an elective event and there is no point placing a woman or her unborn child at significant and unnecessary risk. Syndrome O puts women at risk for miscarriage and later pregnancy complications. Although such decisions may seem arbitrary to many women, physicians are ethically entitled to make these judgments. Since it is impossible to know any particular woman's exact risk prior to an actual pregnancy, I believe that each situation and plan of attack must be individualized. For each couple deciding their options, knowledge is power.

Multiple Gestation Issues

Most triplet and higher order multiple pregnancies are conceived through gonadotropin ovulation induction. At the extreme, the Mc-Caughey septuplets born in 1997 were conceived following hMG treatments. The media concomitantly glamorizes and chastises such events. The details of Mrs. McCaughey's evaluation, fertility treatment regimen, and monitoring were never presented for closer medical scrutiny. The pros and cons of the McCaughey pregnancy outcome, as well as many other less publicized multiple conceptions, continue to spur debate among ethicists, insurance company executives, and fertility care providers.

Since 1980, the number of twin births per year in the United States has increased 74 percent, and the annual number of higher or-der births (triplets or more) has increased 400 percent, according to the March of Dimes and the National Center for Health Statistics. Gonadotropin ovulation induction and IVF treatments have tradi-tionally been considered equally responsible. Before starting a go-nadotropin treatment cycle, the multiple pregnancy possibility should be frankly discussed. The issue should again be raised if more than two developing follicles are found during the monitoring part of the cycle.

There are some overly aggressive fertility specialists who desire pregnancy for their patients at all costs. Fortunately, these doctors are in the minority. Such physicians assert that infertile patients have al-ready been strapped with high expenses and wasted time. And they point to a procedure called selective pregnancy termination that can allow for high-order multiple pregnancy reduction to one or two on-going gestations. Traditionally, the chance of multiple pregnancies conceived from gonadotropin ovulation induction has been cited as 4 to 8 percent, of which about half will be twins.

Ovarian Overstimulation and Hyperstimulation

Overstimulation of the ovaries by gonadotropins and risk for multiple pregnancy go hand in hand. In most cases, such cycles should be canceled, unless an opportunity exists for conversion of the cycle to IVF. If an overstimulated cycle is allowed to proceed through the ovulation induction pathway (i.e., not IVF), there is also an added risk of a medical problem called ovarian hyperstimulation syndrome (OHSS). Carefully monitored, conservative cycles of gonadotropin ovulation induction for growth of one or two follicles should rarely result in significant OHSS. However, when OHSS develops, the ovaries become quite large, and extra fluid (*ascites*) builds up within the abdomen. In severe cases of OHSS, dehydration, poor urine output, and diminished kidney function often occur. The ascites can spread to spaces around the lungs, causing shortness of breath. Excess pressure on deep pelvic veins by the ascites fluid can cause blood clots, thrombophlebitis, and pulmonary emboli. Severe OHSS is a medical emergency and should be managed by a team approach, including the fertility doctor and appropriate critical-care hospital specialists in the fields of renal and pulmonary medicine.

Typical Costs Incurred

Depending on the length of the cycle and the quantity of gonadotropins used, costs can vary considerably. A single 75 unit ampule or vial of recombinant FSH costs about $55 to $70 retail; Serono sells a multidose formulation of FSH that reduces the costs slightly. Currently, the least expensive FSH in the United States is urinary-derived Bravelle, sold by Ferring, which retails for about $35 to $50. There has been some recent downward pressure on prices due to competition among the companies that produce FSH, as well as pharmacies. Although some couples purchase less expensive gonadotropins from outside the United States, this approach can be risky and illegal. Quality assurance may be different outside the United States, and concerns have been raised regarding storage and temperature conditions in certain countries prior to shipment.

Depending on geographic area and insurance participation, the cost of cycle monitoring (ultrasound, hormone levels, physician interpretation, and instruction) can vary from $100 to $500 each day. Intrauterine inseminations add additional cost. Some fertility centers, such as ours, offer global fees for ovulation induction cycle monitoring. In addition, avenues for financing do exist. Since worldwide results with IVF continue to improve each year, couples should carefully compare their options with regard to cost-effectiveness and success. Syndrome O women should also consider the fact that a self-monitored life-management plan of weight loss and exercise costs relatively little and may obviate the need for expensive advanced fertility treatments.

Ovarian Drilling Surgery: Pros and Cons

Gynecology textbooks published as recently as the 1970s were persistent in their discussion of *ovarian wedge resection* as a surgical option for treating ovarian confusion and ovulation disruption. Drs. Stein and Leventhal first introduced this treatment for enlarged, polycystic, nonovulating ovaries in the 1930s, when no medications were available for ovulation induction. Once clomiphene became available in the 1960s, wedge resection was principally advocated as a second-line therapeutic option for clomiphene-resistant patients. Although gonadotropins were used in the 1960s and '70s for ovulation induction, less advanced ultrasound technology and a lack of rapid hormone assays for careful monitoring truly hindered their safety.

Based on current knowledge of ovarian physiology, we suspect that ovarian wedge resection surgery drastically reduced the amount of ovarian androgens being produced. The procedure primarily removed tissue portions containing stromal and theca cells, which are very sensitive to the insulin hormone family and contain the key enzymes for producing androgens. By reducing androgen overload within the ovaries, remaining follicles theoretically would have a chance to grow and develop normally. Of course, wedge resection did nothing to reduce the underlying whole-body metabolic problems associated with Syndrome O. Nevertheless, during the four decades in which the procedure was in vogue, many women successfully ovulated and conceived; in many cases clomiphene was found to be more effective following wedge resection.

However, with ovarian wedge resection there was little standardization regarding how much ovarian tissue needed to be removed. Some doctors still believe that polycystic ovarian disease can be "cured" by removing the ovaries completely. In addressing this issue, Dr. Sam Thatcher writes in his 2000 book *PCOS: The Hidden Epidemic:*

> *PCOS, as has been emphasized over and over throughout this book, is much bigger than the ovary. If it were only the ovary, PCOS should be "cured" by menopause, which it isn't. PCOS of the reproductive years becomes the metabolic syndrome (type 2 diabetes, heart disease, abnormal blood lipid levels) of the post-reproductive years. This is true whether by age or by removal of the ovaries. If removal of the ovaries cured PCOS, women should lose weight after oophorectomy, which is generally not the case.*

Thus, removing ovaries, either in pieces or whole, does not cure Syndrome O, a whole-body problem of insulin overproduction. What should you do if your doctor suggests ovarian wedge resection or surgery to remove your ovaries? Unless there are medical reasons for surgery other than "polycystic" ovaries, it would be worth your time and well-being to seek other opinions.

The Ovarian Drilling Procedure

With the advent of laparoscopy technology, a renewed interest in surgical management of polycystic ovaries came about in the 1980s and '90s. By using focused heat generated by electrocautery or a laser device through laparoscopy instruments, small random holes and craters are drilled into the ovarian surface and underlying connective tissue. Laparoscopy is carried out as an outpatient procedure under general anesthesia, through two or three small openings in the skin, and it typically takes thirty to sixty minutes. Recovery at home usually takes one to three days. It is difficult to know in advance which portions of the ovaries should be targeted. Healthy follicles can typically be destroyed in the process, which could lead to more rapid follicle depletion in older women who may already have limited numbers of working follicles. The most concerning complication relates to possible scar tissue formation, thus adding another potential fertility problem to the mix. If a laparoscopy is planned for other indications, it may be reasonable to include ovarian drilling as part of the procedure. You should discuss complications and potential risks with your doctor as part of informed consent prior to the procedure.

My personal view is that lifestyle and medical management of Syndrome O should preclude the need for surgical intervention. Nevertheless, in selected cases of severe androgen excess and marked resistance to clomiphene or gonadotropin ovulation induction, this procedure may be beneficial. Numerous studies have been published in the past fifteen years demonstrating high rates of ovulation and pregnancy (up to 85 percent) following ovarian drilling. However, as with many journal articles about medical procedures, there is significant potential for publication bias. Many clinical scientists won't take the time or effort to report negative or ineffective findings, especially when their results conflict with previously published articles or the "conventional wisdom."

The Cochrane Collaboration and Library is a well-respected arbiter for evidence-based medicine around the world (www.cochrane. org). In 2001, Dr. C. Farquhar and colleagues at the National Women's Hospital in Auckland, New Zealand, concluded for the *Cochrane Review* that there was no difference in cumulative ongoing pregnancy rates after one year when comparing women treated with ovarian drilling versus ovulation induction with gonadotropins. However, their review of the literature found that multiple gestation rates were significantly lower following ovarian drilling. In one interesting study involving a small number of patients, Drs. U. Muenstermann and J. Kleinstein in Magdeburg, Germany, concluded that six months of medical ovarian and pituitary suppression with leuprolide was equally effective to ovarian drilling. Thus, the debate regarding medical versus surgical therapy continues. Although no one has all the answers, debates like this reflect challenges doctors and their patients around the world must face when considering optimal individualized care for Syndrome O.

IS IT TIME TO CONSIDER *IN VITRO* FERTILIZATION (IVF)?

Technology associated with IVF has made eye-popping advances in the past twenty years. Although many still view IVF treatments as experimental, over 100,000 treatment cycles of IVF were performed in

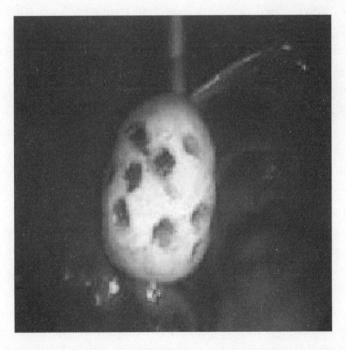

The appearance of an ovary following laproscopic ovarian drilling procedure. Photograph courtesy of Dr. Steve Sawin

the United States in the year 2000 alone, resulting in 25,000 live births of more than 35,000 babies. About 36 percent of live births conceived by IVF were multiple gestations—28 percent of IVF live-births were twins, and 8 percent were triplets or more. Just under 1 percent of all babies born in the United States were conceived through IVF. The utilization of IVF treatment cycles increased 54 percent from 1996 to 2000, and the number of live births increased 73 percent. For the couples who have attained such joy and success following IVF, there was nothing experimental about the babies who joined their families.

There is no absolutely perfect time to consider IVF. During the initial evaluation for infertility, it may become obvious that IVF is necessary for fertility problems other than Syndrome O, such as severe male infertility, fallopian tube disease, or nonrepairable pelvic adhesions. In the setting of Syndrome O infertility, some couples grow weary of month-by-month failures with clomiphene and/or gonadotropin-based ovulation induction regimens. Such couples are usually aware that IVF exists as an option and know that success rates with each cycle of IVF are commonly double or triple the chances of success with ovulation induction. For couples who have not been successful with numerous ovulation induction attempts, the odds with IVF appear infinitely higher from their vantage point.

Experienced professionals in the field of IVF include physicians, registered nurses and nurse practitioners, medical assistants, ultrasound technologists, embryologists, laboratory technologists, patient coordinators, financial counselors, social workers, psychologists, and administrative personnel. Most IVF facilities need a highly specialized team to provide top-notch clinical care and laboratory support. The level of human expertise and technologic advances that must come together in most IVF centers is truly an astonishing phenomenon.

Many different factors influence IVF success rates. The combined efforts of the Centers for Disease Control and the Society for Assisted Reproductive Technology provide information to the public on an annual basis through extensive summaries and clinic-by-clinic details. It is a Herculean effort to compile these statistics, but by the time results are tabulated and made available to the public they are already two to three years out of date. In 2000, a total of 383 clinics reported their outcomes. It appears that a woman's age is the single most important factor determining the chance of a successful live birth with IVF treatment. For women under age thirty-five throughout the United States, 32.8 percent of the 33,453 initiated cycles resulted in a live birth; for women in the thirty-five to thirty-seven age range, 26.7 percent of the 17,284 cycles yielded a live birth. Women of ages thirty-eight to forty had an 18.5 percent live birth rate based on 14,701 initiated cycles; women of ages forty-one or forty-two had a 10.1 percent live birth rate based on 6,118 initiated cycles. The national averages just released for 2001 showed a 1 to 2 percent improvement in success for women under age forty-one, but no significant change for women forty-one and older.

Most IVF practitioners believe that several other important factors provide prognostic information for treatment outcome.

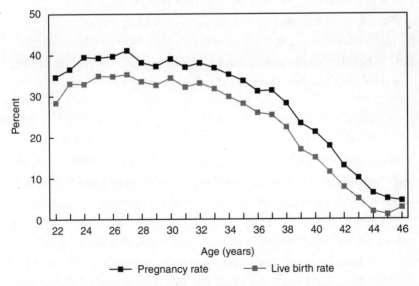

Pregnancy and live birth rates for IVF by age, using fresh, nondonor eggs or embryos, in the year 2000. Graph courtesy of the Centers for Disease Control and the Society for Assisted Reproductive Technology (www.cdc.gov/reproductivehealth/)

Taking the Gamble

I often tell my patients that the probability of IVF success for any specific couple is either zero or 100 percent. It is important to realize that
no two couples are alike and treatment approaches and potential outcomes should be highly individualized. Cost is an important factor for
many couples and different clinics have varying fee structures and financing options. Some facilities offer "shared risk" for IVF, which
provides refunds for certain groups of patients with good prognoses.
There are pros and cons to these types of programs, and they should
be scrutinized carefully. In some states, legislative mandates exist for
IVF insurance coverage. It is no surprise that some of these states (e.g.,
Massachusetts, Rhode Island, Illinois, Maryland, and more recently
New Jersey) have the highest utilization of IVF per capita in the
United States. For example, about 9 percent of IVF cycles in the United
States in 2001 were carried out just in Massachusetts, which has only
2 percent of the nation's population. However, a few studies link uni-
versal IVF coverage to *lower* rates of multiple pregnancy.

Some additional and compassionate expenditures for fertility care
by our society may actually prevent a lot of costly suffering, particularly when high-risk pregnancies and substantial neonatal morbidity
and mortality can be prevented through intelligent IVF care.

The Importance of Patient Health and Fertility

The concept of Syndrome O implies that "all is not perfect" with the
body's glandular internet. Chronic overnourishment and insulin overproduction can interfere with the normal function of virtually every
organ and tissue in the body. The reproductive system is a sensitive
barometer of Syndrome O perturbations, with the health and well-
being of follicles, eggs, and embryos at stake. Since IVF requires both
healthy "seeds and soil," the quality and receptiveness of the uterine
lining (endometrium) to implantation is equally important.

In short, uncontrolled Syndrome O is a negative prognostic indicator for IVF success. With the high emotional stakes, time commitment, and financial burdens associated with IVF, common sense would dictate that strategic insulin-lowering interventions might help. Many patients ask: "How long should I manage my overall health before treatment?" Based on our knowledge of follicle and egg development, a minimum of two to three months of diligent insulin-lowering strategies seems prudent. Taking even more time to become fit also makes sense, especially for women with a BMI over thirty. But there are no quotas on devotion to good health and fertility enhancement.

Unless age and significant metabolic dysfunction cloud the prognosis, prior fertility is seen as a definite positive in IVF treatment circles. In 2000, about 25 percent of the women undergoing IVF in the United States had previously given birth. For those women, their chance of success with IVF was enhanced by 4 to 5 percentage points compared to women without proven fertility. In many clinics, younger women pursuing IVF who had previously given birth and had undergone elective tubal sterilization tend to have the best prognosis. Although many IVF specialists have the impression that prior success with IVF is a plus, national statistics have not been able to clearly evaluate or confirm that opinion.

Responding to Gonadotropins

Controlled stimulation of ovarian follicle growth is the mainstay of effective IVF treatment. Most protocols call for initial suppression of the pituitary gland and ovaries with daily leuprolide injections, followed by concomitant use of gonadotropins. Unless a woman has been treated with gonadotropins previously, it is difficult to know in advance what her ovarian response will be. Most clinicians consider factors such as age, BMI, and infertility diagnosis when deciding on gonadotropin dosing. Some doctors prefer stimulations with only FSH, whereas others prefer a combination of FSH and hMG, which provides some LH in the mix. In the setting of an efficient and well-run IVF laboratory, a target range of eight to fifteen developing follicles during ovarian stimulation seems prudent. Close monitoring with ultrasound and blood hormone levels is a very important component of the gonadotropin-stimulation phase of IVF.

Safe and metabolically controlled ovarian stimulation should be the goal for every patient. Overstimulation of the ovaries can result in inappropriately high numbers of eggs that are possibly not fully mature in their development, nor capable of becoming high-quality embryos. The endometrium may also respond abnormally to excessive stimulation, creating a hostile, nonreceptive environment for embryo implantation. The risk of ovarian hyperstimulation syndrome also rises with increasing numbers of follicles and estrogen levels. Women with Syndrome O are commonly at a higher risk for these problems, since insulin overproduction heightens gonadotropin response.

Some women with Syndrome O may initially respond poorly to gonadotropin stimulation for IVF, since their doctors are trying to be conservative. Cancellation of such cycles can lead to disappointment, frustration, and lost time and money. However, there are no specific medical complications from understimulation. In a subsequent try, the gonadotropin dose will likely be increased. However, this must be done cautiously, as some women are easily prone to convert from underresponders to overresponders.

A growing number of IVF doctors believe that insulin-reducing medications are beneficial to IVF outcome. As of this writing, a few recently published studies support this approach. Insulin-reducing medications are not FDA approved for non-diabetic individuals. Therefore, future studies will be needed to best understand the comparative benefits and risks of both pharmacologic and non-pharmacologic insulin-lowering strategies. Doctors are legally permitted to prescribe drugs for indications other than those specifically approved by the FDA. However, FDA approval for a certain medical indication implies that rigorous studies of safety and efficacy have been carried out and that a panel of experts has carefully scrutinized outcomes. Currently, it appears unlikely that companies manufacturing insulin-lowering medications will invest heavily in studies leading to FDA approval for fertility care usage.

Retrieval of Eggs

Follicle and egg maturation tend to occur together, and the clinical response to gonadotropins plays an important role in egg quality. About thirty-six hours after the injection of HCG—which acts like LH—egg retrieval is scheduled. The number of eggs obtained will correlate with the number of follicles seen on ultrasound. A wide range in egg number, from five to thirty or more, can typically be retrieved from different patients.

Standards of care mandate that the egg retrieval procedure be carried out in a safe, sterile, and well-monitored environment. Over the past ten years there has been a significant shift in the location of IVF facilities from hospitals to private offices. Some have the best of both worlds—i.e., a high-quality office facility on the campus of a large medical center. Ideally, the IVF lab should be adjacent to the procedure room so that eggs are handled expeditiously once retrieved.

There should be no discomfort associated with the egg retrieval procedure, which typically requires twenty to thirty minutes. With the right medications, most patients are drowsy or fall asleep during egg retrieval. Recovery takes one to two hours. Most reputable clinics retain anesthesiologists and/or nurse anesthetists who are experienced with administering and monitoring intravenous sedatives and narcotics. Short-acting medications such as midazolam (Versed) and fentanyl (Sublimaze) provide outstanding conscious sedation during the retrieval and appear very safe for the patient and her eggs. Women with a high BMI often require additional doses of sedation to achieve adequate comfort for the egg retrieval. This issue should be discussed in advance of initiating an IVF cycle. Some anesthesia professionals refuse to administer sedative and narcotic medications to excessively obese individuals in an outpatient setting, mainly because of concerns related to maintaining an airway with adequate oxygen inflow.

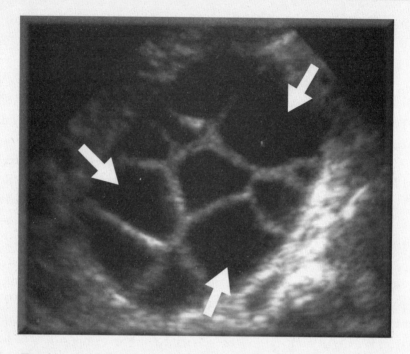

Typical honeycomb ultrasound appearance of the ovary during controlled ovarian stimu-
lation prior to egg retrieval. Each dark area (arrows) represents an individual maturing
follicle containing fluid, with the egg and granulosa cells inside.

During the egg retrieval procedure, a thin needle is placed through
the back of the vagina and into the ovarian follicles via ultrasound
guidance. Gentle suction is applied as the needle enters each follicle
and the fluid and cells from each follicle are aspirated into warm test
tubes kept at body temperature. As each tube of follicular fluid and
cells is collected, the embryologist in the IVF lab should immediately
inspect it. Ultrasound demonstrates the slow collapse of each follicle
as the fluid content is removed and is used as a guide to determine
when the procedure is complete. This technique is much safer and
less invasive than the method of egg retrieval in the 1980s, which required laparoscopy. Occasionally, laparoscopy is still employed in situations when the ovaries are not visible by vaginal ultrasound but it is
not considered optimal, since all follicles cannot be easily seen.

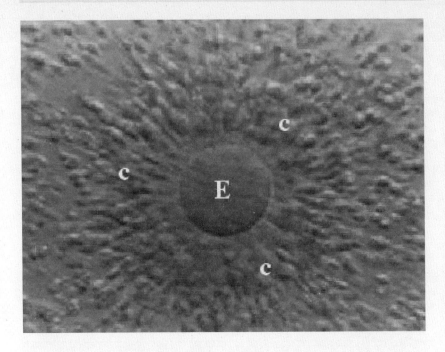

Appearance of the egg (E) soon after retrieval from the follicle. Hundreds of smaller cumulus granulosa cells are attached and/or associated with the egg (c). These cells produce estrogen and a host of other hormones and growth factors that influenced egg development and maturation during the ovulation phase of the cycle.

Introducing Eggs and Sperm

The initial aspect of laboratory IVF involves identifying the eggs in the follicular fluid. An experienced embryologist can empty a tube with follicular fluid and cells into a warmed flat culture dish and identify the microscopic egg in a matter of seconds. Initially, the egg is "born" with hundreds of other surrounding cells—hormone-producing *cumulus* granulosa cells—adjacent to the outer egg shell, or *zona pellucida*. As the embryology team is preparing its work with the eggs, other lab personnel are simultaneously getting the sperm ready to fertilize the egg.

Fertilization of the egg can be achieved through two techniques: the more traditional mixing of one egg with thousands of sperm in a small droplet; or a microinjection of a single sperm directly into the cytoplasm of the egg. The second technique, also known as *intracyto-plasmic sperm injection* (ICSI), has gained a great deal of popularity in recent years. In many IVF labs, it has become the preferred approach. In most cases of male factor infertility, ICSI is strongly recommended, because traditional mixing of eggs with sperm is less likely to achieve fertilization. Other indications for ICSI can include low egg numbers, prior lack of fertilization with traditional IVF, and unexplained infertility. ICSI also provides an opportunity to closely examine the structure and maturity of the eggs soon after retrieval, which can provide important feedback to the clinician who prescribed the gonadotropin induction protocol. Widescale application of ICSI adds a great deal of time and cost to the IVF lab's workload, which may not be practical in very large centers.

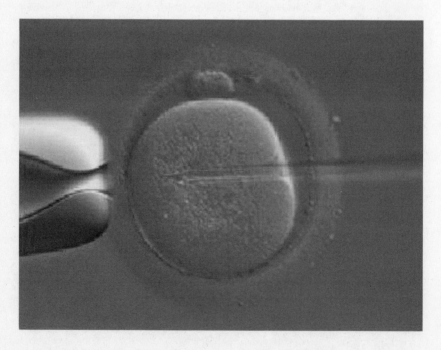

Intracytoplasmic sperm injection (ICSI) of a mature egg. Under the microscope, a holding device (left) keeps the egg steady as a sharp glass needle injects a single sperm into the jelly-like cytoplasm inside the egg.

Safety issues and pregnancy outcomes continue to be monitored closely by the world's community of IVF specialists. The first ten years of ICSI results appear very reassuring, based on healthy outcomes for thousands of babies conceived by this approach. Certain ICSI cases truly push the limits of IVF technology by utilizing very sparse or underdeveloped numbers of sperm. In some of these cases, paternal genetic abnormalities may bias some of the research and conclusions regarding the actual ICSI technique.

Embryo Quality

Maternal age and health are often powerful predictors of embryo viability. Although shoddy clinical and laboratory techniques can cloud the picture, younger and fertile women tend to produce healthier, genetically normal embryos that are more likely to implant in the uterus.

Healthy, high-quality embryos undergo remarkable developmental changes in their first seven days of life. Within six to twelve hours of introducing sperm to the eggs, either by traditional IVF or ICSI, the first discrete evidence of normal fertilization is the presence of two nuclei. One nucleus contains one set of chromosomes and genes from the mother; the other nucleus contains a single set of the father's genetic material. Together, the two sets of chromosomes merge and align themselves within a single nucleus of the original egg cell to form a unique new embryonic heredity. Gradually, fertilized eggs undergo cellular division over a forty-eight-hour period, changing from one cell to balls of eight cells. Pictures from the microscope only capture the two-dimensional aspects of these astonishing three-dimensional entities. Each cell within a developing embryo is called a *blastomere* and contains all of the genetic material of the future child. When embryos split at this stage, they function as clones and form the basis for monozygotic, or identical, twins. Most IVF clinics transfer embryos to the uterus three days after retrieval, typically at the six- to eight-cell stage.

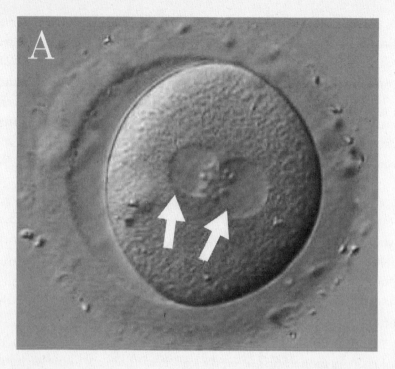

A fertilized egg under the microscope in the IVF lab. The earliest evidence of normal fertilization is the appearance of "kissing nuclei" (arrows), also called the 2PN stage.

Embryo Transfer and Implantation

Early human embryos are the seeds of life and are handled with extreme care, particularly for their journey to and potential germination within the uterus. In this regard, the IVF team prepares the embryos in the lab, while the clinical team has prepared the patient for an optimal intrauterine environment. In almost all instances, progesterone supplementation has been started the day of the egg retrieval, with the intent on continuing it through the first ten to twelve weeks of pregnancy. Progesterone is needed as an important supplement following egg retrieval, since a high percentage of the follicles' cells were removed. Some debate continues over whether daily intramuscular injections or twice daily vaginal administration of progesterone is optimal; our clinic has a bias toward the older but more uncomfortable intramuscular method. We also supplement the post-retrieval phase of treatment with oral estrogen to help sustain endometrial receptivity.

The actual embryo transfer procedure involves the loading of embryos by the embryologist into a thin, flexible catheter, which is then introduced by the clinician into the uterine cavity. Embryo transfer is a painless procedure, which takes just a few minutes. However, it is such a crucial part of the whole IVF process that we utilize abdominal ultrasound by an experienced sonographer to help visualize and guide the precise location of the catheter. Patients are asked to drink some water ahead of time since a full bladder helps visualize the uterus and catheter on ultrasound. Often it is possible to see a tiny fluid wave at the precise time that the embryos are nudged into the uterus. This is very reassuring to the patient and the IVF team. Published studies indicate that ultrasound-guided embryo transfers enhance implantation and pregnancy rates.

For most couples ages thirty-five and under, it seems most reasonable to transfer just one or two healthy embryos to the uterus. At this time, it is much more common in the United States to transfer two embryos. For some patients, it may be appropriate to transfer three or more embryos, but this must be carried out on an individualized basis and with appropriate informed consent. Increasingly, IVF clinics and government-sponsored health units outside the United States are advocating single embryo transfers.

IVF lab and clinical specialists are constantly striving to improve ways to enhance embryo quality, as well as implantation rates. One laboratory technique, termed *assisted hatching,* may yield more efficient embryo implantation by creating a small opening in the zona pellucida, or outer eggshell, of the embryo. Two techniques exist for assisted hatching of embryos under the microscope: 1) directing a dilute solution of acid at a specific spot in the zona pellucida; or 2) firing a laser beam at the zona pellucida. This manipulation may permit more efficient embryo growth, expansion, and hatching. Experimental techniques that may have future application include co-culture of embryos with maternal endometrial cells, noninvasive embryo culture diagnostics, and enhancement of culture media with specific growth factors or hormones.

Extended Culture

In many IVF labs around the world, extended culture of embryos to the *blastocyst* stage is carried out. As embryos continue to develop, their metabolic requirements change, particularly after the eight-cell stage. Under proper culture conditions, eight-cell embryos should divide and undergo *compaction,* a process that makes discrete cell borders of the blastomeres impossible to delineate. These embryonic structures are called *morulae.* Within one or two more days, healthy morulae usually divide and blossom into more advanced embryonic organisms called *blastocysts.*

Blastocyst culture technology is the subject of much investigation and debate, even beyond IVF treatment circles. The inner cell mass (ICM) of the blastocyst is a cluster of cells that are destined to develop into a fetus. They are commonly called stem cells, and they have the potential to develop into virtually every organ and tissue type. Cells in the outer cell mass (OCM) are also called *trophectoderm cells,* and they are the progenitors of the placenta. Although much remains to be learned about the biology of these human embryos, healthy blastocysts containing robust ICM and OCM have higher rates of implantation compared to eight-cell embryos. It makes sense that this would be the case, since many eight-cell embryos are incapable of developing into blastocysts. Thus, day 3 transfer might provide an advantage to average-appearing eight-cell embryos, where certain uterine factors might enhance their development and chance of implantation.

Couples desiring single embryo transfers would probably have the best odds of success by utilizing extended culture technology to identify a single outstanding-appearing blastocyst. Not all IVF clinics offer this option. For couples preferring transfer of two embryos, there is no proof that waiting for blastocyst formation is advantageous. Currently, pregnancy rates tend to be quite similar when comparing double embryo transfer at day 3 versus day 5 or 6 (i.e., time of blastocyst formation). However, the chance of twins is higher with two embryo blastocyst transfers. Because of extra work in the IVF lab, routine blastocyst culture technology also requires additional resources and cost.

Embryo Freezing

At this time, our IVF facility prefers to transfer the healthiest appearing eight-cell embryos to the uterus on day 3, with ongoing observation of remaining embryos in extended culture conditions. For extra embryos that are able to develop into blastocysts, cryopreservation (freezing) is recommended. This meticulous procedure requires gradual changes in culture media and slow temperature decline in a special chamber. After several hours, the cryopreserved embryos are placed individually in a tank containing extremely cold liquid nitrogen. Cryopreservation offers several important advantages. First, cryopreserved blastocysts can be utilized in subsequent cycles if a fresh embryo transfer was unsuccessful. Also, cryopreserved blastocysts can be thawed and transferred months to years later, if a previously successful couple desires more children. Finally, cryopreservation of lower quality, poorly developed embryos can be avoided.

During a twenty-four-month period in our facility, from 2000 to 2002, blastocyst technology and cryopreservation provided our patients with an 81 percent cumulative clinical pregnancy rate and a 66 percent cumulative birth rate. These results, which included patients of all ages and diagnoses, were presented at the 2002 meeting of the American Society for Reproductive Medicine, and are similar to successes observed in some other clinics. Cryopreservation technology continues to improve, with a newer and more efficient freezing process called *vitrification* being evaluated at the current time.

For patients considered at high risk for ovarian hyperstimulation syndrome (OHSS), cryopreservation has significant benefits. Generally, OHSS worsens in a setting of early pregnancy and avoidance of embryo transfer can offset that risk. Usually, such patients (who can include a number of insulin-overproducing Syndrome O women) produce high numbers of eggs and embryos and tend to be younger in age. As such, the likelihood of achieving significant blastocyst number and quality is high, and the survivability of such cryopreserved embryos can approach 60 to 80 percent. In the study cited above from our center, the ongoing pregnancy rate from thawed blastocysts was 45 percent, matching or exceeding results for fresh embryo transfers in many clinics.

SHOP TILL YOU DROP

IVF facilities come in all different shapes and sizes. Currently there are about 450 centers that perform IVF in the United States. They range in performing as few as five to ten cycles, or as many as three thousand each year. In the year 2000, centers that performed more than two hundred cycles tended to have slightly better pregnancy rates. Success rates are highly dependent on the types of patients that are getting treatment. Couples with better prognoses sometimes demand IVF treatment early in the process, even when less aggressive and less expensive measures would potentially work. On the other hand, some doctors push unsuspecting couples into IVF prematurely.

Smaller clinics may provide highly personalized and professional care, which may or may not be more costly. Highly successful large clinics were often small successful clinics just a few years earlier. Clinics with "big names" are sometimes resting on their past laurels, whereas "lesser-name," high-quality facilities often attract informed couples who have carefully done their research. Published statistics by the CDC (www.cdc.gov/reproductivehealth/) are typically two to three years out of date and can only provide a guide for the general standard of care around the country. Paying attention to the buzz in your community regarding the professionalism of particular centers may be useful, even if it is not a particularly scientific approach.

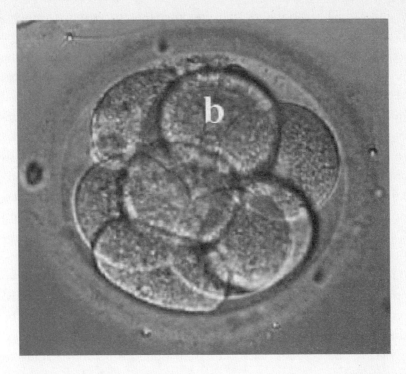

A normal-appearing human embryo under the microscope in the IVF lab, at the eight-cell stage. Each embryonic cell is called a blastomere (b).

WHEN NOTHING SEEMS TO WORK

Not every couple benefits from the treatment options and techno-logic advances of modern fertility care. This is a sad truth, but many couples face this realization with strength and dignity. There may be specific explanations for lack of success with IVF, such as poor egg, sperm, and/or embryo quality diagnosed during the treatment. In other cases the presence of excellent-quality embryos may point to an underlying problem in the endometrium, which could be inhibiting implantation. Careful evaluation (or re-evaluation) of the uterine cavity by hysteroscopy may have value in these instances.

Abnormal responses of the endometrium to estrogen, progesterone, and the insulin family of hormones may have a role in unexplained and repetitive IVF implantation failures. I have had the
privilege of working with one expert in the field of endometrial receptivity, Dr. Harvey Kliman at Yale University, who has found that
many women exhibit delayed development of the uterine glands during the time of embryo implantation. Although this problem appears
to be more common among infertile women with endometriosis
and/or unexplained infertility, it underscores the potential susceptibility of the female reproductive system to subtle hormone and metabolic swings. Dr. Bruce Lessey, at the Greenville Hospital in South
Carolina, is another recognized expert in assessing endometrial abnormalities. His team has investigated problems associated with production of integrin molecules, which may be vital for early embryo
attachment to the endometrium. Application of human endometrial
research to problems of clinical infertility continue to be explored by
these and other dedicated investigators.

Many couples seek second or third opinions before deciding to
stop treatments. For women affected by Syndrome O, this could be an
important option, since practitioners view problems of insulin overproduction and ovulation disruption from different perspectives. Unlike women who may have no obvious explanation for their repetitive
lack of success, women with Syndrome O have options to explore for
reducing overnourishment and improving insulin sensitivity in their
bodies. I have witnessed many women transform their prognosis and
treatment success by effective, long-term strategic personal planning
and intervention.

How many times is it reasonable to try IVF? Generally, after three
or four attempts at a good clinic, the chance of success in subsequent
cycles tends to drop. A lot depends on a woman's age and what has
been learned in prior cycles about embryo quality. Ultimately, if IVF
doesn't work for you, it may be appropriate to explore other family-
building options, such as adoption, donor egg, donor embryo, or surrogacy. These are all expensive and potentially complex avenues to
travel. Depending on your fortitude, determination, creativity, and the

size of your pocketbook, they may or may not be the right choices for you.

KEEPING YOUR CHIN UP: KEY MOTIVATIONAL POINTS

- A number of key discoveries and technologic developments over the past seventy-five to one hundred years have converged to provide constantly improving odds of success for millions of couples seeking fertility care in the United States and around the world.
- The discovery and development of gonadotropin hormones FSH, LH, and HCG for pharmacologic use has resulted in the birth of countless babies over the past forty years. Until recently, gonadotropins were purified and prepared only from the urine of menopausal and pregnant women.
- Low-dose gonadotropin administration is often used for ovulation induction, particularly in situations where clomiphene has not been successful. In this setting, it is absolutely required that gonadotropin usage be carefully monitored by ultrasound and blood hormone levels.
- High-risk multiple pregnancies can result from the overzealous, unmonitored use of gonadotropins. A medical complication called ovarian hyperstimulation syndrome (OHSS) can lead to a severe medical emergency affecting many organ systems.
- Ovarian drilling by laparoscopy may have a role in reducing ovarian androgen production, thus allowing conservative attempts at ovulation induction. Ovarian surgery doesn't heal the whole-body problems associated with Syndrome O.
- Making the decision to pursue IVF treatment is a big step for many couples. Every year, IVF results in about 1 percent of the babies born throughout the United States. Thousands of couples find success with IVF each year.
- Successful IVF clinics utilize an expert and professional team of clinicians, lab personnel, and administrative support. Al-

though there are never guarantees, the majority of couples pursuing IVF will eventually be successful. Age, embryo quality, and overall good health are important prognostic factors.

- Intelligent IVF utilizes a combination of compassion, ethics, individualized care, conservative embryo transfer, and good common sense. Syndrome O women can improve their odds by carrying out a plan to eliminate overnourishment and reducing insulin overproduction.

- Smart consumers of both general fertility and IVF care should evaluate the pros and cons of each center in their geographic vicinity. Second or third opinions are often prudent before making the decision to stop treatment.

- Although it can be difficult to cope with unsuccessful treatments, persistence does pay off for many couples. Fertility care is often a private matter. However, consider taking advantage of support systems that likely exist in your family, circle of friends, colleagues, and house of worship. You are not alone in your quest to build a family.

SIX

SYNDROME O AND MISCARRIAGE

ADDRESSING THE PROBLEM

"It was like I was pushed off a cliff," one of my patients reflected about her recent miscarriage. "We had tried so hard to get pregnant. All those blood tests and ultrasounds. And then there were hours of hopes and prayers. I felt like something precious died when I saw the ultrasound screen that day."

There are few soothing words to be offered when a pregnancy loss is first identified. As an objective and sympathetic practitioner, I find this to be the saddest news I have to give to my patients. The best I can hope to achieve under such circumstances is to work toward providing an explanation. Unfortunately, in many instances, no easy explanation can be found.

For many couples it can help to intellectualize the sad experience. Thinking about and hearing potential causes for pregnancy loss often creates a sense of empowerment and positive thinking for the future. "After all," stated one of my favorite patients, "at least we were able to get pregnant." As it turns out, that intuitive reasoning is correct.

Most women who achieve one pregnancy are able to conceive again, even if the pregnancy ended in miscarriage.

I often evaluate patients in my practice who have suffered either single or multiple losses and usually deal primarily with women who have had first-trimester miscarriages (i.e., earlier than the thirteenth week of pregnancy). In many cases it is necessary to reconstruct the events and tests that were done prior to the loss, when the patient was under someone else's care. For patients who are followed closely by a doctor from the time of conception, it is easier to piece together what happened. Luckily, for patients who are followed in this manner, it is rare for pregnancy loss emergencies (i.e., heavy bleeding, cramping, passing of tissue, pain) to occur unexpectedly.

The presence of polycystic ovaries and insulin resistance has been linked to miscarriage for many years. Syndrome O, particularly when uncontrolled, places women at higher risk for pregnancy loss, as well as later complications. The insulin family of hormones affects all aspects of female reproduction, including the follicles and eggs, embryo implantation, and the development of the embryo, fetus, and placenta. Maternal blood flow to and from the developing fetus can be hampered by insulin overproduction. In a recent patient fact sheet titled "Weight and Fertility," the American Society for Reproductive Medicine stated definitively that obesity is linked to miscarriage. Metabolic dysfunction should always be considered a potential factor in any woman who suffers a pregnancy loss.

What causes miscarriage? When attempting to identify the underlying cause(s) of miscarriage, three main clinical categories of early pregnancy loss can be observed: fetal demise, empty gestational sac (i.e., "blighted ovum"), or chemical pregnancy loss. Each of these are described separately below.

Fetal Demise

By the sixth week of pregnancy, or about two weeks after a missed menstrual period, sensitive ultrasound can usually detect a tiny fetus, measuring just 2 to 5 millimeters, along with prominent motion of the fetal heart. Adjacent to the fetus is a small, round structure called the yolk sac, which is thought to produce stem cells for the fetus. From this point in the pregnancy, weekly ultrasounds should demonstrate growth of the fetus, ongoing cardiac activity, and overall growth of the uterus and pregnancy sac. After demonstration of fetal growth and heart motion, the prognosis is excellent. About 95 percent of such pregnancies will continue to develop normally in younger women. Women over age forty have a less optimistic prognosis, with a 20 percent loss rate even after fetal heart motion had previously been seen. For pregnancies that stop developing, there is the sad observation of a small fetus without heart activity. In most of these cases, there were no clinical symptoms. Textbooks refer to this as a "missed abortion," probably because in the era before ultrasound it was not possible to know that the pregnancy had stopped developing.

Empty Gestational Sac

In this setting, an intrauterine pregnancy sac can be easily visualized by ultrasound, but there is no fetus present. This situation usually reflects an inability of the inner cell mass of the blastocyst to grow and develop properly. If only the outer cell mass develops, cells of the blastocyst can still attach to the uterine lining and grow for several weeks. A nonviable pregnancy with an empty gestational sac can be diagnosed as early as two to three weeks after a missed menstrual period.

Chemical Pregnancy Loss

Many pregnancies fail to develop beyond the earliest phases of implantation. For several days or more, HCG—produced by the embryonic placental cells—can be detected in the mother's blood. However, those levels quickly fall, suggesting the absence of an ongoing pregnancy. Ultrasound may demonstrate a thickened lining within the uterus, but usually no evident pregnancy sac. In some instances, HCG levels plateau, or rise slowly in an inappropriate manner. This scenario raises the possibility of a pregnancy located outside of the uterus, called an ectopic pregnancy. Ectopic pregnancy in the fallopian tube is a potentially dangerous and life-threatening problem, treated by laparoscopy, or medically with injections of methotrexate. It is strongly recommended that all patients with abnormally rising HCG levels be followed closely until the pregnancy test becomes negative.

SEEDS AND SOIL

Although all females of the animal kingdom produce eggs, only mammals have evolved the ability to nourish their embryos and unborn offspring within their bodies. In practically every mammalian species, the uterus provides a fertile environment for embryo implantation and fetal growth—like soil for a seed. Problems with either seedling embryos or the uterine lining in which they must germinate will often create hazards for an early pregnancy.

Age and Eggs

Abnormalities of the embryo can often be preordained, based on the genetic or metabolic makeup of the egg or sperm prior to conception. More often, the health and well-being of the egg is the principal issue. In the final days before ovulation, eggs change their genetic makeup by undergoing an important process called *meiosis*. During meiosis, the egg must literally push out half of its chromosomes to make room for a new set of chromosomes from the sperm. Within the egg, this process of chromosome realignment can result in errors, leading to a retained chromosome, a missing chromosome (whole or part), or even more complications. Genetics specialists refer to this problem as *chromosome nondisjunction*. One of the most well-studied genetic abnormalities in humans—trisomy 21, or Down syndrome—usually involves a chromosome nondisjunction error in the egg. In this setting, an extra chromosome #21 remains in the egg during meiosis, prior to fertilization.

Many other chromosome errors can also occur during meiosis, resulting in a conception containing three copies of one or more chromosomes (trisomy), or just one copy of one or more chromosomes (monosomy). It is estimated that about 50 percent of genetically abnormal pregnancy losses are due to chromosomal trisomy. Most of these errors result in early pregnancy loss, usually in the first trimester. Some conceptions are not even identified as clinical pregnancies, since they fail to develop at the embryonic stage. It is not known what factors within the developing egg and follicle lead to nondisjunction chromosome events, as well as other errors in egg development. However, advancing maternal age is directly linked to the likelihood of such problems. Clinicians have known for many years that Down syndrome, as one example, is more prone to occur as a function of maternal age. Many other genetic abnormalities within the egg demonstrate a similar age-related association.

Women of any age can produce eggs with chromosomal abnormalities. In fact, about 80 percent of Down syndrome pregnancies occur in women *under* the age of thirty-five. Likewise, many other genetic problems can occur in younger women, although the prevalence is lower. One common genetic abnormality leading to miscarriage—Turner syndrome—is not related to maternal age and may actually be more common in younger women. In most cases of Turner syndrome, the embryo is lacking one of the sex chromosomes, resulting in a set of 45 chromosomes including one X chromosome (designated by genetics specialists as 45,X). There is no specific evidence that Syndrome O places women at higher risk for producing genetically abnormal eggs. However, as an egg undergoes meiosis just prior to ovulation, the right hormone environment within the follicle is critical for egg development.

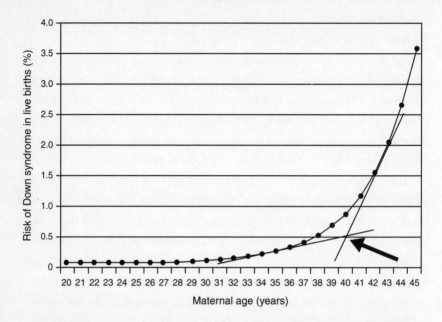

Increased risk of Down syndrome (trisomy 21) as a function of maternal age. Many other chromosome abnormalities in the egg reflect a similar age association, with a significant inflection in the curve around age 39 to 40 (arrow). Graph courtesy of American Academy of Family Physicians

OPTIONS FOR GENETIC TESTING

The contribution of genetic abnormalities to the overall incidence of pregnancy loss is quite high and may account for 50 to 75 percent of all first-trimester miscarriages. As with IVF, new technologies have given practitioners an array of testing options, some of which are mainstream and others which are currently in the development phase.

Since an abnormal chromosome count is such a common factor contributing to miscarriage, it is the policy in our practice to recommend testing of pregnancy-loss tissue whenever possible. For patients, this requires a minor procedure called *dilatation and evacuation* (D&E), which can be performed under mild general anesthesia or conscious sedation in an outpatient surgery center. Briefly, the cervix is gently dilated and a suction catheter removes the tissue. Once tissue is obtained, it is immediately transported to a lab that specializes in tissue growth and chromosome analysis. A time period of two to four weeks may be required for final results from the lab. In general, tissue obtained at the time of D&E has a better chance of yielding genetic information compared to tissue passed at home during spontaneous miscarriage. Genetic information is also more likely to be found in pregnancy losses of more advanced gestational age. In cases of chemical pregnancies or very early empty sac losses, tissue analysis is usually unrevealing, and D&E probably won't be helpful.

However, laboratory analysis of pregnancy loss tissue for chromosome count is not always revealing or accurate. In some cases, cells from the pregnancy cannot grow in the lab, making the analysis impossible. Very often, the lab will issue a report demonstrating normal 46,XX chromosomes (i.e., a normal female). This is often nondiagnostic, since the cells analyzed may have derived from the mother's uterine lining, not the pregnancy itself. This was proven in an important study published in 1999 by Drs. Karen Bell, Peter Van Deerlin, and myself at the University of Pennsylvania. A re-evaluation of fourteen archival pregnancy loss specimens by more sophisticated genetic and DNA analyses found that four of the tissues (29 percent) had been incorrectly characterized as normal female 46,XX. These patients had been told that their pregnancy losses were "genetically normal."

It is common to recommend chromosome testing for prospective parents who have suffered pregnancy loss. Lymphocytes (white blood cells) can be extracted from a single tube of blood, and the chromosomes can be analyzed closely. In 2 to 5 percent of pregnancy loss cases, either parent may harbor a chromosome rearrangement that places future conceptions at risk for an imbalanced complement of chromosomes. In very rare instances, a parental chromosome problem could signify that a couple will never achieve a normal pregnancy. Although this is troubling information for a couple to absorb, it does allow them to pursue donor egg or sperm options, and/or to rethink their need for contraception to prevent future miscarriages.

THE FUTURE OF GENETIC TESTING

Assisted reproduction is gradually being applied to the problem of repeated pregnancy loss. A technique called *preimplantation genetic diagnosis* (PGD) allows for detailed chromosome analysis of embryos before they are transferred into the uterus. Remarkably, a single blastomere cell can be removed from an eight-cell embryo without harming the embryo. The blastomere is then stained with multicolor markers for each of the twenty-three different chromosomes by a technique called *fluorescent in situ hybridization* (FISH). Those embryos that contain extra or missing copies of a particular chromosome would be considered nonviable. Older women and/or women with a history of pregnancy loss are often found to have high numbers of chromosomally abnormal embryos when they undergo IVF and PGD. In some cases, however, a few normal embryos are found, which can dramatically improve the prognosis for a genetically normal pregnancy. Some researchers in the field believe that PGD techniques will eventually be applied to all IVF cases. At the present time, only a few labs across the country have the expertise to utilize these techniques.

Chromosome testing does not provide the universal picture regarding the impact of genetics on pregnancy development. Counting chromosomes is like viewing the hazy outlines of the earth's continents from outer space. Specific genes within chromosomes—like the earth's rivers, mountains, and cities—determine the details of an organism's destiny. Scientists are just beginning to apply a wealth of genetic knowledge to the field of human reproduction, and specific genes necessary for normal embryo and pregnancy development are gradually being identified. Perhaps most fascinating for women with Syndrome O is the gradual assessment of early pregnancy genes controlled by the insulin family of hormones.

The Uterine Factor

To uncover structures that could interfere with an implanting or growing pregnancy, it is important to understand the uterine cavity. Problems with the uterus include polyps, fibroids, and adhesions (Asherman's syndrome), which even if small, could interfere with an otherwise normal pregnancy. Asherman's syndrome refers to chronic scarring inside the uterus, and is a potential complication of uterine curettage, or D&E, and may not be recognized until years after the procedure. It is more likely to occur if post-procedure infection or retained tissue was a complicating event. Women can also be born with uterine problems, such as a uterine septum, a "heart-shaped" (bicornuate) uterus, or a uterus that has a narrow cavity on the inside. Of these abnormalities, the uterine septum is most commonly associated with early pregnancy loss. A uterine septum is a fibrous band of tissue dividing the uterine cavity, which lacks important blood vessels needed for a developing pregnancy.

For diagnosing such problems, doctors commonly use an X-ray test that is called a hysterosalpingogram (HSG). Other noninvasive imaging tests like ultrasound and/or MRI can also help evaluate the anatomy of the uterus. Treatment of certain uterine problems, like a septum, require hysteroscopy and laparoscopy to correct. During a thirty- to sixty-minute procedure under general anesthesia, the septum is incised, which leads to the creation of a completely normal uterine cavity and a reduction in miscarriage risk. More complex cases of large uterine fibroids or congenital uterine abnormalities may require an abdominal (laparotomy) approach.

The glandular tissue lining the uterus, the endometrium, is truly the soil in which an embryo must germinate. Other problems throughout the body associated with inflammation, infection, or abnormal immunity could interfere with embryo-endometrial interactions. The association of Syndrome O, metabolic dysfunction, and obesity with higher rates of miscarriage implicates the insulin family of hormones as key regulators of early pregnancy.

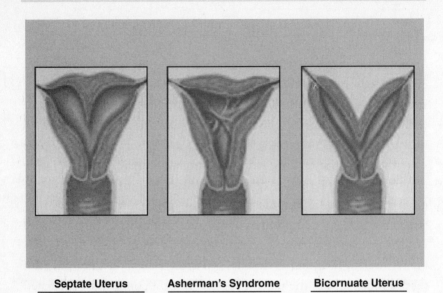

Septate Uterus	**Asherman's Syndrome**	**Bicornuate Uterus**
Wedge of fibrous tissue dividing uterine cavity.	Adhesions (band-like formations) crossing the lining of the uterus.	Incomplete uniting of uterus.

An artist's rendering of three types of uterine abnormalities diagnosed by hysterosalpingogram. Septate uterus and Asherman's syndrome are associated with pregnancy loss, whereas bicornuate uterus is more commonly associated with preterm labor and delivery. Figure courtesy of Ohio State University reproductive medicine division

THE INSULIN FAMILY: THERE FROM THE BEGINNING

Human reproduction cannot progress normally without insulin, or without a number of binding proteins and insulin relatives, known as *insulin-like growth factors* (IGFs). The pathways and intricacies of the insulin hormone family have become increasingly fascinating, as scientists apply new technologies for probing insulin and IGF actions within follicles, eggs, embryos, and the endometrium. The insulin hormone family has profound effects on fetal growth and the subsequent outcome of pregnancy. Overnourishment and insulin overproduction can interfere with pregnancy at every step. Therefore, the insulin hormone family must be tightly controlled and normally functioning during early development, or reproduction will fail.

Follicles and Eggs

Although thousands of eggs lie dormant for many years, once follicles begin to grow, eggs within those follicles become directly affected by a woman's metabolic state. In conjunction with FSH and LH, insulin and IGFs instruct ovarian theca cells to convert LDL-cholesterol to androgens. This is carried out through instructions to the genes that code for enzyme proteins in the theca cells. Once androgens are produced, granulosa cells carry out another set of enzyme instructions to produce estrogen. The insulin family is vital to this process within the developing follicle. Excess ovarian androgens stimulated by the insulin family interfere with healthy follicle and egg development. Over-nourishment and insulin overproduction further impair follicle growth and egg development, leading to ovarian confusion and ovulation disruption. Even if ovulation is achieved, optimally healthy eggs may not be released.

Embryos and Blastocysts

Early embryos also need insulin and IGFs, but only in amounts that are consistent with the mother's heredity, not her current overnourished environment. Many researchers have demonstrated that mammalian embryos contain the receptors and active genes necessary to respond to insulin and IGFs. It is likely that the insulin hormone family is vital for regulating embryo metabolism and growth. Before implantation, an embryo is bathed in secretions from the fallopian tubes and uterus, which contain maternal hormones. As soon as implantation is initiated, the embryo is exposed to nutrients and hormones in the mother's bloodstream.

In animal studies, embryos cultured with excess insulin or IGFs undergo abnormal development and, in some cases, premature cell death. Dr. Kelle Moley's research group at Washington University in St. Louis has found that embryos exposed to high concentrations of insulin or IGF-1 are much less likely to undergo healthy blastocyst development. The cells of the blastocyst most profoundly affected are the inner cell mass (ICM) that is destined to become the fetus. For Syndrome O women, this observation means that miscarriages would often occur at the earliest time of implantation, leading to chemical pregnancy losses or complete implantation failure. Alternatively, embryos exposed to toxic levels of insulin or IGF-1 could lead to ICM-depleted blastocysts and empty gestational sac pregnancy losses.

The developing placenta requires specific levels of insulin and related growth factors. Placental cells known as *trophoblasts* start as stem cells derived from the outer cell mass, or *trophectoderm,* of the blastocyst. Without healthy trophoblasts, implantation cannot occur. Many hormones, including the insulin family, signal trophoblasts to initiate attachment and invasion of the endometrium as part of the implantation process. Some trophoblasts synthesize scaffolding proteins to anchor the placenta, while other trophoblasts carefully and systematically invade small blood vessels in the uterus to provide oxygen and nutrients from the mother's bloodstream.

Numerous researchers have determined that IGFs are produced by the placenta and that these hormones will regulate placental growth. When the mother is overnourished, imbalances in the placental response to insulin and IGFs often lead to later pregnancy complications, including abnormal fetal growth and maternal diabetes. If the maternal insulin system is uncontrolled, fetal death can occur at any gestational age. It has been known by the medical community for many years that poorly controlled diabetes dramatically increases risk of fetal and placental abnormalities, with pregnancy loss as an unfortunate consequence.

The Endometrium

When healthy plant seeds are first introduced to soil, germination and seedling growth will only occur if the soil contains a balance of nutrients and essential elements. Too much fertilizer in the soil could actually be toxic to the growing plant and its root structure. The insulin family of hormones can be viewed as fertilizer for the endometrium, stimulating production of essential proteins and substances required for a developing pregnancy. The endometrium is susceptible to hormones from other glands (for example, estrogen, progesterone, androgens, and insulin), as well as insulin-like growth factors and binding proteins produced locally in the scaffold-like connective tissue cells.

Embryo implantation and germination within the endometrium invokes a complex and rapid sequence of cellular and molecular events. Although it occurs easily and efficiently in many fertile women, implantation is considered the major limiting factor for couples who are undergoing fertility care. For women who achieve pregnancy yet suffer pregnancy loss, increased attention has been devoted to the endometrium as a source of problems. From a research perspective, the human endometrium is a unique tissue, and studies in lab animals do not really provide insight to the human situation. Dr. Linda Guidice at Stanford University is widely recognized for leading a research group that has identified specific IGFs and IGF-binding proteins critical to human endometrial function. A balance of these proteins is believed to be necessary for normal implantation and subsequent healthy pregnancy progression.

Glandular internet communication between the endometrium and placenta is vital for all phases of pregnancy. The placenta contains a delicate root structure called *villi* that provides exchange of oxygen, nutrients, hormones, antibodies, and even waste products between the separated bloodstreams of mother and fetus. The villi are buried deep within the tissues and blood vessels of the uterus, leading to a network of communication between the mother's bloodstream, the endometrium, the placenta, and the fetal circulation.

Clinical Implications

Can reduction in insulin overproduction both prior to and after conception prevent miscarriages? Recent studies examining the impact of the insulin-reducing drug metformin (Glucophage) on women with Syndrome O suggest the answer is a resounding "yes." Although clinical investigators are just beginning to design and publish meaningful studies, early results are encouraging. Dr. C. J. Glueck and his clinical research group at the Jewish Hospital in Cincinnati, Ohio, were the first to publish their results in 2001. Using a study involving ten women, their findings showed that before metformin was introduced, the women had twenty-two previous pregnancies with sixteen first-trimester spontaneous abortions (73 percent). While taking metformin, these same ten women had six normal live births (60 percent), one spontaneous abortion (10 percent), and three normal ongoing pregnancies (30 percent). Although this study examined a small number of women, the effect of metformin in reducing miscarriage was highly statistically significant. Furthermore, there was no evidence that metformin was harmful to the women or babies born in this study.

A second study published in 2002 by Dr. D. J. Jakubowicz and colleagues in Venezuela confirmed the findings of Dr. Glueck's group. Although retrospective in its design, this study compared miscarriage rates in women with excess insulin, some who had taken metformin during pregnancy and some who had not. Sixty-five women taking metformin had a pregnancy loss rate of 8.8 percent, whereas the control group (women not taking metformin) had a 41.9 percent rate of miscarriage. These findings were highly statistically significant and suggested that one insulin-lowering medication strategy might be highly effective for all women who overproduce insulin.

These studies raise some important questions. Can life-management strategies that promote sustained insulin reduction be just as effective as drugs like metformin? With hundreds of thousands of Syndrome O women working toward pregnancy, is it safe and cost-effective to treat all of these women with metformin? Would a combination of nonpharmacologic and pharmacologic approaches be most effective? What is the impact of medications such as metformin on fetal organ development and subsequent infant and adult metabolism? Along with many colleagues in the fertility and pregnancy loss fields, we are paying close attention to the study results and ongoing debates regarding use of insulin-lowering medications for miscarriage prevention and the promotion of healthy pregnancies.

Despite cautious enthusiasm regarding the published results, some Internet sites already scream out the "virtues" of using metformin before and during pregnancy. I advocate diligent and disciplined life-management strategies, as described in depth in chapters 8 and 9. For diabetes prevention, life-management strategies have actually been proven to be superior to metformin. Most important, whenever medications are promoted to benefit pregnant women, prudence is the highest virtue. For this issue, the results of larger prospective studies are definitely needed.

CHECKING OUT YOUR THYROID

It is possible that not enough attention is paid to the function of the thyroid gland in maintaining fertility and healthy pregnancy. The incidence of thyroid dysfunction—principally, underactivity of the gland—appears to be a growing problem around the world. Years ago, an underactive thyroid was linked with goiter and iodine deficiency. More recently, we've learned that the thyroid can be disrupted by factors such as elevated cholesterol, insulin overproduction, obesity, and autoimmune damage. It is easy to screen for thyroid function with a blood test for the pituitary hormone called *thyroid stimulating hormone* (TSH). Elevated levels of TSH in the blood suggest thyroid underactivity (i.e., hypothyroidism), whereas a depressed TSH indicates thyroid overactivity (hyperthyroidism). In reproductive-age women, hypothyroidism is common and has been linked to infertility and miscarriage. All reproductive-age women should be screened for hypothyroidism, and hormone replacement treatment is strongly advocated. Fortunately, a once daily oral thyroid hormone called levothyroxine (Synthroid, Levothroid, Levoxyl, Unithroid) is considered safe and desirable for nonpregnant and pregnant women alike. Many pregnant women taking thyroid hormone require increasing amounts of medication as their pregnancy progresses. This is likely due to changing metabolic needs and weight gain. A simple TSH test carried out several times throughout the pregnancy could prevent many pregnancy losses and risk to the developing fetus.

A Newer Diagnosis Emerges: Thrombophilia

Blood is the substance of life. The cellular components of blood include oxygen-carrying red blood cells and white blood cells for fighting infection and inflammation. Platelets are derived from cells in the bone marrow and work as the first line of defense in promoting blood clot formation following injuries to tissues and blood vessels. Dissolved in the liquid component of blood—the plasma—are a large number of proteins and enzymes that both create and destroy blood clots. Clotted blood within an artery or vein is called a *thrombus*. Dangerous blood clots often occur within the coronary arteries, lungs, or deep veins of the legs. Spots of injury or inflammation within arteries or veins can lead to life-threatening blood clots. Any imbalance in the clotting system that inappropriately promotes thrombus formation is called *thrombophilia* (from the Latin for "clot loving").

Many proteins that create clots throughout the body are produced in the liver. The discovery of the clotting cascade—the sequence of protein and enzyme reactions required for clot production—was one of the greatest discoveries in medical science. The body must also have a mechanism to dissolve clots at the proper time. The liver produces many potent enzymes, such as plasminogen, that are activated at the site of clots when it is safe for them to be removed. Cells lining blood vessels, platelets, and other tissues produce proteins that either enhance or impede thrombus formation. The body must constantly maintain a balance in pro-coagulant and anticoagulant activity at every location. This balance is extremely important at the site in the uterus where an embryo is implanting. From the earliest time of implantation, embryonic trophoblasts of the placenta invade and remodel the mother's blood vessels, allowing a vital exchange of oxygen and nutrients. It is here, deep within the uterus, that a life-giving equilibrium between anticlotting and pro-clotting factors must occur.

Thrombophilia has been increasingly associated with pregnancy loss. Placental villi float in lakes of maternal blood, like water lilies in a pond. The trophoblasts lining the villi produce anticoagulant substances to help maintain a constant flow of blood through these maternal lakes. If the wrong pro-coagulant substances disturb this delicate balance, inappropriate clots can occur in the blood surrounding the villi. In such a setting, an otherwise normal pregnancy can literally be strangulated by a lack of oxygen and nutrient exchange.

Both inherited and acquired problems can contribute to thrombophilia and subsequently to increased risk for pregnancy loss. In many situations, a combination of factors leading to thrombophilia increases miscarriage risk. The list of acquired and inherited causes of thrombophilia has grown rapidly, and includes the following:

Pro-coagulant Antibodies

The most extensively studied substances related to pregnancy loss and later complications are the antiphospholipid antibodies (APLA). Many theories exist to explain why people develop these antibodies, but the precise reason is unknown. About 5 to 10 percent of women with repeated pregnancy losses test positive for APLA. Common names for APLA include the anticardiolipin antibody and the lupus anticoagulant. In women who have had previous miscarriages and test

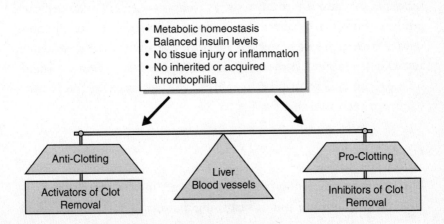

positive for APLA, treatment during subsequent pregnancies greatly reduces the chances of another miscarriage.

Estimates of the incidence of elevated APLA in the general population range from 2 to 20 percent. APLA can induce clotting in the maternal blood surrounding the placental villi, but not typically in other locations. Some pregnant women can develop the more severe "APLA syndrome," which leads to significant complications in later pregnancy, including poor fetal growth, fetal death, maternal hypertension, and thrombosis in the uteroplacental circulation. Some women may also be at risk later in life for thrombotic events, but the exact risk isn't known.

Some fertility clinics test all prospective pregnant women for anti-cardiolipin and lupus anticoagulant, with the rationale that APLA-positive patients should be offered the option for treatment when a pregnancy occurs. It is not yet possible to determine which APLA-positive patients would benefit most from knowing this information prior to pregnancy. A common treatment regimen during pregnancy uses a daily combination of minidose aspirin and a single subcutaneous injection of low molecular weight heparin (Fragmin, Lovenox). Low molecular weight heparin is considered safe. It does not cross from the mother's blood to the fetus, and it may prevent inappropriate clot formation within the placental implantation site and maternal blood vessels surrounding the villi.

Couples should be cautious about pregnancy loss centers that offer expensive and unproven tests, as well as treatments that are unproven. Some practitioners treat pregnancy loss patients empirically with aspirin and low molecular heparin, even when no identifiable antibodies are found. Although it is difficult to endorse this as a wide-scale practice, there may be benefits to this approach in specific instances of recurrent miscarriage.

Inherited Thrombophilia

With so many different proteins and enzymes involved in clot formation and dissolution, it is not surprising that many different inherited disorders exist. Modern molecular biology techniques have identified specific mutations and rearrangements in coagulation-related genes that lead to thrombophilia. Individuals exhibiting abnormal clotting may test positive for markers in their DNA, and often these genetic problems are found within related family members. Clinical scientists are just scratching the surface to understand the impact familial thrombophilia has on pregnancy. Even more uncertain is the role of specific treatments designed to minimize clot formation in such individuals. Since pregnancy itself greatly enhances liver production of clotting factors, a genetic predisposition for thrombophilia could lead to an enhanced risk of life-threatening clots elsewhere in the body. Birth control pills stimulate the liver in a similar fashion, and in this case are usually contraindicated. Direct consultation with a hematologist is strongly recommended for any reproductive-age woman found to have a personal or family history of thrombophilia.

One well-studied cause of inherited thrombophilia is a rearrangement in the gene coding for clotting Factor V, called the Leiden mutation. Individuals carrying one or both gene copies of Factor V Leiden are at increased risk for thrombotic medical problems throughout the body. Some biologists have theorized that Factor V Leiden has been a relatively silent mutation in the history of mankind until recently, when other environmental factors, such as overnourishment and inactivity, have contributed to risk of thrombophilia. Some clinical researchers have found an association linking Factor V Leiden to miscarriage; other studies refute this point. It is possible that certain individuals with Factor V Leiden may be at increased risk for pregnancy loss when other thrombophilic factors, such as APLA or insulin overproduction, are also present. Widespread genetic testing for different inherited thrombophilias, although just requiring a DNA test from a single tube of blood, is expensive. Such testing may not be cost-effective unless a specific personal or family history warrants evaluation.

Insulin and Thrombophilia

Insulin resistance, obesity, and insulin overproduction have been strongly linked with a predisposition for thrombosis. Millions of type 2 diabetic individuals are known to be at significantly higher risk for coronary artery obstruction and vascular disease. Metabolic dysfunction profoundly affects the delicate balance of pro-coagulant and anti-coagulant systems throughout the body. Given the unique nature of blood circulation at the site of early pregnancy, it is not surprising that Syndrome O women are at particular risk for thrombophilia.

A great deal of attention has been paid to a protein called *plasminogen activator inhibitor type one* (PAI-1), and the role it may play in linking insulin overproduction to thrombophilia. PAI-1 controls how fast clots can be dissolved, and excess levels of PAI-1 will interfere with the body's efficiency in breaking up clots. Insulin overproduction has been closely linked to PAI-1 overproduction throughout the body. Too much PAI-1 can tip the scales toward thrombophilia. At the delicate site of pregnancy implantation, PAI-1 is produced both in the endometrium and placenta, suggesting its important role in regulating blood flow and clotting.

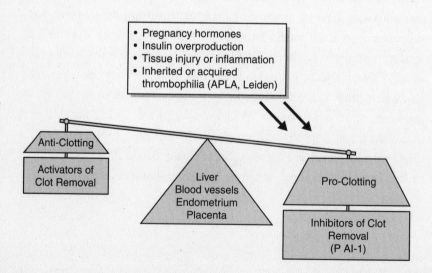

Important studies by Dr. Charles J. Lockwood and colleagues at New York University and Yale University have identified several key proteins involved in endometrial hemostasis and clot removal. They have found that PAI-1 is significantly regulated in the endometrial stroma by estrogen, progesterone, and other hormonal growth factors. Although numerous pro-coagulant and anticoagulant proteins are produced and regulated by endometrial and trophoblast cells, excess PAI-1 could markedly disrupt blood flow and normal placental function.

Metformin significantly lowers PAI-1 levels in Syndrome O women who previously suffered miscarriages, suggesting that PAI-1 is a marker of pregnancies at risk. It is likely that markers like PAI-1 can be improved prior to conception with insulin-lowering strategies (chapters 8 and 9), and that risk of miscarriage and later pregnancy complications could be minimized.

GOOD FORTUNE AND COMMON SENSE: KEY MOTIVATIONAL POINTS

Most couples do not expect the heartbreak of miscarriage when they first achieve a pregnancy. However, it is a sad reality of human repro-

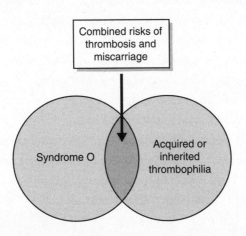

duction. Fortunately, there are both explanations and mechanisms for prevention that could help thousands of couples each year. Although having an explanation for miscarriage from your doctor may aid in the grieving process, pregnancy loss can be a very emotionally trying experience. Every couple deals with loss differently, and it is likely that men and women will exhibit different emotional responses. Most doctors are able to refer couples to professional counselors and/or support groups for assistance.

If Syndrome O is affecting your metabolic and reproductive systems, insulin-lowering strategies are a must. Developing a strategic plan now—at least several months before attempting pregnancy—could be all the medicine you need for a normal and successful outcome.

The vastly popular book *What to Expect When You're Expecting* starts out with the exclamation "Congratulations—and welcome to your pregnancy!" For many women this is appropriate, and there is little reason for them to be concerned. However, women who suffer with infertility, Syndrome O, or a history of one or more pregnancy losses probably need to be more circumspect. A healthy pregnancy requires some thought, action, and prayer long before the time of conception.

Some key points to consider are:

- The emotional turmoil of pregnancy loss can be tempered by carrying out a compassionate and thoughtful investigation of all possible contributing factors. Although answers are not always forthcoming, the prognosis for subsequently achieving a normal pregnancy is good for most women.
- Clinical categories of first-trimester pregnancy loss include fetal demise, empty gestational sac ("blighted ovum"), and chemical pregnancy loss. Ectopic pregnancy should be suspected if HCG levels demonstrate a plateau or are rising at an inappropriate rate. This can be dangerous and should be monitored closely by your doctor.

- The integrity of the chromosomes within the egg is one of the most significant issues surrounding miscarriage. Errors during meiosis lead to imbalances in chromosome number, including trisomy and monosomy of any chromosome. Many chromosome abnormalities such as Down syndrome, or trisomy 21, occur more frequently as women become older.

- Uterine factors, such as fibroids, polyps, and adhesions, can prevent normal pregnancy progression, particularly if they are located close to the site of implantation. A congenital uterine septum contributes to some cases of pregnancy loss. Diagnosis and treatment usually involves therapeutic hysteroscopy.

- Metabolic dysfunction and insulin overproduction should always be considered as potential factors in any woman who suffers a pregnancy loss. The insulin family of hormones, including insulin, IGFs, and IGF-binding proteins, orchestrate normal physiology within the follicle, developing egg, early embryo, and blastocyst. The endometrium responds to the insulin family in order to permit normal embryo-uterine cross talk and implantation.

- Metformin shows promise in reducing miscarriage rates in women with Syndrome O. Larger, well-designed studies are needed to assess the risks and benefits of medication-based protocols. In the meantime, women with Syndrome O should implement safe and cost-effective personal insulin-lowering strategies.

- Thrombophilia ("clot loving") refers to an increasingly important problem of excessive blood clotting, which may place some women at higher risk for miscarriage. Acquired thrombophilia, as caused by antiphospholipid antibodies, may necessitate treatment with minidose aspirin and low molecular weight heparin. Clinical scientists continue to identify new causes of inherited and acquired thrombophilia.

- Syndrome O adds a superimposed risk to thrombophilia, particularly during pregnancy. Insulin overproduction exacerbates thrombophilia by increasing the body's production of pro-clotting proteins like PAI-1. Insulin-lowering strategies will help restore the delicate balance of clotting and blood flow throughout the body and most especially within the uterus and placenta of a developing pregnancy.

SEVEN

SYNDROME O AND RISKY PREGNANCIES

Tina's Sadness

Modern medicine seemed to fail Tina when she needed it most. When I discharged her from our care in the third month of her pregnancy, there were lots of hugs, kisses, and fanfare in our office. Tina's first cycle of *in vitro* fertilization (IVF) had been successful, and she was pregnant with twins. All seemed well with the ultrasound at twelve weeks of pregnancy, so she was now transferring her care to a well-respected group of obstetricians. Three months later, a funeral was held. Tina's perfectly formed babies were born much too early, even for the modern miracles of neonatal medicine to give them a chance.

Unbeknownst to Tina and her obstetricians, her growing uterus probably began contracting, and her cervix began dilating weeks ahead of schedule. A routine ultrasound performed at nineteen weeks of pregnancy did not detect any problems. Tina continued to go about her daily routine. A few days before the babies were born, Tina began to feel pelvic pressure, but her doctors reassured her. As the pressure in her vagina increased significantly one night, her only choice was to rush to the emergency room. By that time, doctors found her cervix almost fully dilated and, despite some last-minute heroic efforts to prevent delivery, the babies would not wait. At twenty-two weeks gestation and weighing ¾ pound each, there was nothing more the doctors or nurses could do. A short time after the birth, the babies—a boy and a girl—were wrapped gently in blankets and died peacefully in Tina's arms.

Tina is a tenacious young woman with Syndrome O. Since her teenage years she suffered with irregular and heavy menstrual periods, obesity, and unwanted facial and body hair. Doctors never adequately explained things to Tina and usually prescribed birth control pills to control her menstrual cycles. Then she met Ted, eventually got married, and came to our practice for fertility care. Unbeknownst to them, Ted's sperm count was quite low and different options for treatment were discussed. After several unsuccessful attempts of ovulation induction and artificial insemination, the couple turned to IVF. Their pregnancy outcome was beyond belief to Tina, Ted, and all who cared about them. Could Tina's Syndrome O have been a factor? Are there studies linking overnourishment, insulin overproduction, or obesity to the escalating rates of premature labor and delivery? In order to help Syndrome O women like Tina, it is time to explore the evidence.

The Scope of the Problem

Preterm labor and delivery is a scourge on our society, affecting countless families every year. According to the March of Dimes, about 12 percent, or one in eight of pregnancies in the United States deliver prematurely—i.e., before the thirty-seventh completed week of gestation. Fortunately, modern neonatal medicine can save and treat the majority of babies born prematurely, but medical complications can persist for years in preterm infants and children. While you might have read about babies who are born early and do very well, the truth is that those babies are the exceptions. Babies who are born preterm are at a very high risk for developing neurological, breathing, and digestive problems within the first few days of life. Unfortunately, they are also at risk for problems later in their lives. Simply put, the earlier in a pregnancy a child is born, the more health problems that child is likely to have. Survival is not even possible prior to twenty-four completed weeks of pregnancy.

With all of the scientific advancements we have made, why are one in eight pregnant women in the United States suffering from preterm labor and possible premature birth? Despite the fanciest technology and newest biochemical testing available at thousands of hospitals throughout the land, we have barely made a dent in our ability to prevent and predict preterm labor. Experts in the field of high-risk pregnancies have blamed many underlying factors for the persistently rising rate of this problem. Most of these factors are environmental and related to the mother's health, suggesting that in a perfect world most cases of preterm labor and birth could be prevented. Obvious bad habits like smoking, alcohol, and illicit drug use during pregnancy raise the risk substantially. A great deal of attention has also focused on untreated infections, including venereal diseases (for example, chlamydia and gonorrhea), group B *streptococcus,* and excessive bacterial colonization of the vagina and cervix (bacterial vaginosis). Many bacterial strains release by-products that cause inflammation in the cervix, uterus, and fetal membranes, leading to softening and dilatation of the cervix and uterine contractions.

Is Fertility Care to Blame?

Fertility care has been widely criticized for contributing substantially to preterm infant morbidity and mortality. The media often adds to this perception by sensationalizing the wonders of high-order multiple births, which almost always deliver quite prematurely. Some overly aggressive fertility care providers have added to the risk, but this issue should be kept in perspective. In 2000, analysis of U.S. IVF statistics indicate that a total of 1,762 women delivered triplets or higher, representing just 0.04 percent of all live births in the United

States. Twin deliveries following IVF were more common, number-
ing 6,500, or 0.16 percent of all U.S. births. Overall, IVF twins and
triplets contribute just 2 percent to the group of pregnant women at
high risk for preterm birth. Ovulation induction treatments may add
a similar number of at-risk women, but statistics for this group are not
tabulated or known precisely. The point is that even if conservative
fertility treatments resulted in singleton pregnancies 100 percent of
the time, the rate of preterm labor and delivery in the United States
would hardly change.

Premature Births Related to Obesity

For a number of years it was believed that overweight women rarely
had premature births, since the fetus was well nourished and protected *in utero*. More recent scientific analysis challenges this impression. Dr. Richard Naeye, a highly esteemed pathologist at Penn
State–Hershey Medical Center, wrote a landmark article in 1990 entitled "Maternal body weight and pregnancy outcome," published in
the *American Journal of Clinical Nutrition*. In this, he reported an analysis of more than 56,000 pregnancies in which he correlated perinatal
mortality rates with maternal weight. He noted that the risk of newborn death rose dramatically—more than 225 percent—in obese
women compared to thin women, and the increased mortality was
due in large part to preterm delivery prior to thirty-one weeks of
pregnancy. A high percentage of the preterm deliveries demonstrated
evidence of infection and inflammation in the placentae, which
could have been caused by pathologic vaginal organisms and/or early
dilatation of the cervix. Other contributing factors to neonatal mortality included maternal diabetes, being over age thirty-five, congenital abnormalities in the fetus, and twin pregnancies. Fertility care was
hardly a factor in the 1980s when this cohort of pregnant women was
analyzed.

Another landmark article published in the *New England Journal of
Medicine* in 1998 further examined the relationship between pre-
pregnancy weight and risk of adverse outcomes. The study reviewed

more than 167,000 pregnancies in Sweden—a country considered one of the healthiest in the world—in 1992 and 1993, with Dr. Sven Cnattingius as the lead author. Quite unlike the situation in the United States, only 6.2 percent of the Swedish women had a pre-pregnancy body mass index (BMI) greater than 30. Preterm labor and delivery is also much less frequent in Sweden as compared to the United States.

This study only included pregnancies with a single child. Amongst Swedish women pregnant for the first time, a BMI over 30 increased the probability of a preterm birth before thirty-two weeks by 55 to 60 percent, compared to women with a BMI less than 30. More disturbing, the incidence of late fetal death increased more than 100 percent in women with a BMI greater than 30, suggesting some significant problems affecting blood flow to and nourishment of the developing fetus.

An editorial that accompanied the article suggested that "there may be something inherently hostile in the intrauterine environment of obese pregnant women" and that obese women should be considered at increased risk for serious perinatal outcomes. It further proposed that "the possibility of minimizing risk to the fetuses carried by obese pregnant women through interventions such as altered maternal weight gain or dietary supplementation should be studied."

Specialists in obstetrics and high-risk pregnancies know that many different factors can link obesity and insulin overproduction to preterm birth and poor neonatal outcomes. Overweight and obese women, including many with Syndrome O, often have high blood pressure prior to and during pregnancy, underlying vascular disease, disturbances in pro-clotting pathways, elevated lipid and cholesterol levels, worsening glucose intolerance and diabetes, and dysfunction of fetal growth and development. There are also specific issues regarding the mode of delivery, with larger babies of diabetic women requiring cesarean section more frequently.

Although difficult to design and carry out, interventional studies prior to pregnancy are needed to help guide women affected by overnourishment and insulin overproduction. Until the results of such studies come along, it seems logical that Syndrome O women might enhance the health of their pregnancies and unborn children by carrying out pre-conception life-management strategies.

Taking a Stand

Government agencies such as the National Institutes of Health and the U.S. Surgeon General's Office have addressed the overt risks to pregnancy caused by obesity and overnourishment. The March of Dimes has had a long track record of devoting their resources and research dollars to diagnosis and treatment of preterm labor and premature birth. The organization estimates the annual cost of care related to premature labor and delivery to be more than $11 billion. Research dollars devoted to the problem are 1 to 2 percent of that amount.

In 2002, the March of Dimes Task Force on Nutrition and Optimal Human Development released their findings, which stated that: "Birth defects, premature birth, and other severe health problems in tomorrow's babies are linked to the soaring rates of obesity among women of childbearing age." According to Dr. Richard Deckelbaum, a professor of nutrition at Columbia University in New York who chaired the task force, "Weight before pregnancy matters much more than people realize, even health professionals. For the moms, there are serious complications such as gestational diabetes, dangerously high blood pressure, and hospitalization; and for the babies, prematurity, serious birth defects, and other severe problems. And when these babies grow up, they are more likely to suffer from obesity, cardiovascular disease, diabetes, and other health problems. Obesity is particularly dangerous for women of childbearing age because it creates a life cycle of serious problems that can be passed from generation to generation."

New Beginnings for Tina

It took great courage for Tina to attempt another pregnancy. She was devastated by the loss of her twins, and she felt a combination of

enormous guilt and remorse. Although Syndrome O was not the primary reason Tina had needed IVF, she recognized the impact it could
have had on her prior pregnancy experience. After the losses, her life
became one of great introspection and re-evaluation. Tina became
determined to make some significant changes in her life, and she
worked hard to modify her nutrition and activity and stress levels. After several months, she felt better about herself and her future.

With a strong marriage and the support of her family, Tina again
pursued IVF. She had very cautious optimism related to her prior success in getting pregnant. Unfortunately, the next time around with
IVF wasn't successful. She garnered the strength to try once more,
and with the transfer of just two embryos, Tina again was carrying
twins. This time, everyone vowed to be on heightened alert.

Toward the end of the first trimester, vaginal ultrasound revealed a
curious phenomenon—Tina's cervix was already starting to shorten,
pointing to a high risk of premature delivery. Given her prior history,
she was immediately referred to the high-risk specialists at our medical center, who debated about Tina's medical management. Based on
her prior history and clear evidence of cervical change in the early
going of this pregnancy, the decision was made to place a *cerclage,* or
stitch, within the muscular portion of her cervix. Tina was also told
to stay off her feet as much as possible.

At nineteen weeks of pregnancy, Tina's cervix had stretched out
almost 100 percent and started to dilate. Although the high-risk
specialists were at a loss to provide any additional treatment, Tina was
admitted to the hospital for observation. The uterine monitor
demonstrated contractions off and on. At twenty-two weeks she was
warned about the high chance of delivery, and the fact that nothing
could be done to save the babies. She held firm in her resolve. At
twenty-five weeks the pediatric team was alerted, but Tina stayed
camped out in her hospital bed in the high-risk maternity unit.

There was practically a victory celebration among the staff on that
hospital unit when Tina delivered her babies at twenty-nine weeks.
She had been treated with glucocorticoids (steroids) to help advance
the babies' lung maturity. Her newborn infants—a boy and a girl—

were tiny but strong at birth. Incredible advances in neonatal medicine kept them alive, and they did very well in the neonatal intensive-care unit. Tina and Ted took home two healthy babies, thus a new beginning for their family.

Despite improving technology in the fields of ultrasound, uterine monitoring, and newer biochemical screening tests, modern medical science has not made a dent in the incidence of preterm labor and delivery. If anything, the problem is worsening, both in cost and emotional turmoil. Treatments for preterm labor have hardly changed since I was a resident in obstetrics twenty years ago—bedrest, intravenous fluids, ongoing monitoring of uterine contractions, exams for cervical stretching and dilating, and combinations of moderately risky drugs to relax the uterine muscle. Perhaps more resources should be devoted to maternal health prior to pregnancy as a way to prevent this escalating problem.

HIGH-PRESSURE PREGNANCIES

Although volumes continue to be written about hypertensive disorders of pregnancy, diseases with names like *preeclampsia, eclampsia,* and *toxemia* still cause many sleepless nights among the world's obstetricians and high-risk pregnancy specialists. This is with good reason, since the American College of Obstetricians and Gynecologists (ACOG) estimates that hypertensive disease occurs in about 12 to 22 percent of pregnancies and is responsible for 18 percent of maternal deaths in the United States. Gestational hypertension—defined as abnormally high blood pressure—can occur as early as the second trimester and is diagnosed when a woman with previously normal blood pressure consistently develops readings greater than 140/90. Many pregnant women who are hypertensive, particularly in their first pregnancy, can develop a more severe multi-organ disease called preeclampsia. Worsening preeclampsia, with or without eclamptic seizures, is a major contributor to maternal and newborn morbidity and mortality.

Almost overnight, a seemingly healthy pregnancy can change to one of extreme risk for mother and unborn child. All health professionals caring for pregnant women have witnessed this familiar and rapid sequence of events: blood pressure moving from slightly high to extremely high; worsening edema ("puffiness") concomitant with significant weight gain; headaches with or without strange visual changes; abdominal pain; and *proteinuria*—when the kidneys spill protein from the blood into the urine. In short order the liver, red blood cells, and the body's clotting systems can also go into a tailspin. As blood vessels feeding the uterus and placenta become more constricted due to hypertension, the fetus may demonstrate overt signs of distress. Even more concerning, the placenta can separate from its attachment site (placental abruption), causing profound bleeding and extreme risk to mother and fetus.

If the heart rate pattern on the fetal monitor is considered reassuring, buying some time for fetal growth and development is important at a very premature gestational age. Mother and fetus are generally hospitalized in a high-risk unit and observed closely. An intravenous drug called magnesium sulfate has been the mainstay of therapy for worsening preeclampsia, along with specific blood pressure–lowering drugs. One key role for these treatments is the avoidance of seizures, or fullblown eclampsia. Maternal and fetal death can rapidly occur in the setting of eclampsia. There is only one known treatment for unremitting preeclampsia—delivery of the child. Often this must take place rapidly, via emergency cesarean section and multispecialty intensive-care monitoring.

The Scope of the Problem

Most specialists in obstetrics and maternal-fetal medicine now accept the viewpoint that the hypertensive diseases of pregnancy constitute a complex syndrome, associated with a variety of underlying risk factors. Like Syndrome O, hypertensive disorders of pregnancy represent a whole-body problem affecting women's reproductive organs, blood vessels, liver, and clotting systems. Very compelling evidence now suggests that metabolic dysfunction, insulin overproduction, and hypertensive disease during pregnancy are closely linked. According to the recent report by the U.S. Surgeon General, maternal obesity raises the risk of developing gestational hypertensive disease tenfold.

Are certain hypertensive complications of pregnancy preventable? To the extent that overnourishment, insulin overproduction, and obesity may be controllable prior to pregnancy, the answer may be yes. However, like many other diseases that exist in our society, an inherited predisposition for preeclampsia cannot be reversed. Likewise, certain underlying disorders affecting the vascular and clotting systems add substantial risk to the development of gestational hyperten-

OBESITY AND PREGNANCY
FROM THE U.S. SURGEON GENERAL'S WEB SITE:
WWW.SURGEONGENERAL.GOV/TOPICS/OBESITY/
CALLTOACTION/FACT_CONSEQUENCES.HTM

- Obesity during pregnancy is associated with increased risk of death of both the baby and the mother and increases the risk of maternal high blood pressure tenfold.
- In addition to many other complications, women who are obese during pregnancy are more likely to have gestational diabetes and problems with labor and delivery.
- Infants born to women who are obese during pregnancy are more likely to be high birth weight and, therefore, may face a higher rate of cesarean section delivery and low blood sugar (which can be associated with brain damage and seizures).
- Obesity during pregnancy is associated with an increased risk of birth defects, particularly neural tube defects such as spina bifida.

sion, and these factors may not be easily identifiable prior to pregnancy. Nevertheless, a careful appraisal of newer information regarding insulin resistance and pregnancy-related hypertension may add fuel to the notion of prevention for many women.

Insulin and Hypertension in Pregnancy

In the late 1980s and 1990s, articles began to appear linking insulin overproduction to hypertensive diseases of pregnancy. In 1988, Nobel laureate Dr. Rosalyn Yalow and colleagues wrote in the *American Journal of Medicine* that many hypertensive women they evaluated in the last trimester had marked insulin overproduction, particularly after a glucose challenge test.

It is known that pregnancy itself can worsen insulin resistance, and preconception insulin overproduction exacerbates the problem significantly. Women who have hypertension prior to getting pregnant are also at much higher risk. Drs. Caren Solomon and Ellen Seely of Harvard Medical School published a compelling and thorough review in 2001 in the journal *Hypertension,* in which many research studies were cited linking insulin overproduction to hypertensive diseases of pregnancy. Their conclusions are particularly relevant to women with Syndrome O. They note that pregnancy hypertension and preeclampsia might have been identified earlier in women who were known to be insulin-resistant. In addition, they advise two important strategies that women can institute before getting pregnant: 1) increased physical activity (an important way to improve insulin sensitivity); and 2) increased fiber in the diet (with carbohydrates like most fruits and vegetables that release sugar slowly into the bloodstream). Unless told otherwise by their doctor, most pregnant women can also safely implement these recommendations.

The Uterine Battleground

Many scientists believe that the invasive movements of placental trophoblasts deep into the uterus during the early weeks of pregnancy predetermine the risk of hypertensive disease later in pregnancy. Pathologists who have closely studied the "placental bed" of the uterus—the place where the placenta was attached—have found a relative inability of trophoblasts to invade and modify many of the mother's blood vessels in that location. As a result, the blood vessels remain constricted and less able to supply nourishment and oxygen to the placenta and fetus. Some of these blood vessels have significant abnormal fatty deposits appearing quite similar to atherosclerosis under the microscope. As the pregnancy grows and blood flow demands increase, a cascade of hormonal events is thought to take place, which raises the mother's blood pressure. This is the body's way to compensate for the constricted, atherotic uterine vessels. For a while, this provides better blood flow to the uterus and placenta. Larger babies and placentae, as seen in diabetic pregnancies, cause even higher demand for uterine blood flow. Eventually, a hypertensive crisis can develop, placing the mother and fetus in a precarious state.

We do not know to what extent the mother's preconception metabolic state affects trophoblast-uterine interaction, but the strong link found between Syndrome O and miscarriage suggests a vital connection. Furthermore, once pregnancy occurs, no medical treatments have proven successful in preventing the onset of gestational hypertension or preeclampsia. In 2002, Dr. S. Bjercke and colleagues from the University of Oslo in Norway published an important study in *Gynecologic and Obstetric Investigation*. They found that women with polycystic ovaries were much more likely than other women to have both gestational hypertension and diabetes. Those mothers also had larger babies with a much higher need for cesarean section delivery and intensive-care monitoring after delivery.

When determining risk factors for disease, doctors like to measure blood levels of hormones, proteins, and other substances. Scientific data has associated insulin resistance with hypertensive disease of pregnancy because of similarities in blood markers related to insulin overproduction. These include elevations in pro-clotting proteins such as PAI-1 (discussed in previous chapter) and triglycerides and decreased liver production of the insulin-sensitive protein SHBG.

Disruptions in the insulin family of hormones, as found with Syndrome O, affect the uterine environment and vascular system, which consequently impact implantation and the health of an ongoing pregnancy.

Several recent retrospective studies have linked gestational hypertension, preterm birth, and low birthweight babies with a 70 to 260 percent higher risk of maternal coronary artery disease later in life. It seems likely that for many women, both Syndrome O and pregnancy-related hypertensive disorders are part of a lifelong metabolic continuum that encompasses the reproductive years and beyond.

A Not-So-Sweet Ending: Gestational Diabetes

Gestational diabetes is a unique metabolic derangement to women in their third trimester of pregnancy, which usually abates soon after delivery. However, longitudinal studies in the 1960s and '70s found that women who had gestational diabetes were at much higher risk than other women for developing type 2 diabetes later in life. This suggested that women with gestational diabetes had a profound underlying metabolic risk. With the epidemics of obesity, overnourishment, and metabolic syndrome rising in the general population during the past thirty years, it is no surprise that gestational diabetes has become a major complicating problem of pregnancy. According to the American College of Obstetricians and Gynecologists, gestational diabetes affects 2 to 5 percent of all pregnancies—80,000 to 200,000—in the United States each year. Countless other pregnant women have clear evidence of insulin overproduction and obesity, yet do not test positive for diabetes. As already discussed, other severe pregnancy problems can occur separately in overweight women, or concomitantly with gestational diabetes.

Making the Diagnosis

Because gestational diabetes is so common, it is recommended that all pregnant women be screened for this diagnosis in the early part of the third trimester. The screening test is easy, done by asking the patient to drink a small amount of sweet cola containing 50 grams (200 calories) of glucose, followed by a single blood test one hour later. If the blood test reveals a high glucose value, then the patient is advised to undergo a lengthier glucose tolerance test several days later. This is carried out with a 100-gram (400 calories) sugar load early in the morning, after a fasting blood test for glucose is performed. Additional blood samples are then drawn at one, two, and three hours after the 100 grams of sugar are ingested. In order to pass the three-hour glucose tolerance test, the fasting blood glucose level should be under 95 milligrams/deciliter, along with post-sugar load blood levels under 180, 155, and 140 milligrams/deciliter at one, two, and three hours respectively. The diagnosis of gestational diabetes is made if two or more blood levels exceed those cutoffs. An abnormality in one value may warrant re-screening one to two weeks later, since it suggests glucose intolerance, a pre-diabetic state.

For Syndrome O women, preconception and early pregnancy testing may also be warranted. In our practice, all Syndrome O women are screened for diabetes with a two-hour glucose tolerance test before starting fertility treatments. We also assess fasting insulin, triglycerides, and cholesterol as other indicators of insulin overproduction. With increasing awareness about insulin resistance in women with Syndrome O and polycystic ovaries, reproductive endocrinologists may be the physicians most frequently diagnosing insulin overproduction, diabetes, and glucose intolerance in young women. As with every other fertility and pregnancy problem associated with insulin overproduction, the same approach is vital in preventing gestational diabetes: controlling metabolism by eliminating overnourishment and controlling weight through increased activity and fitness.

Monitoring Metabolic Progress

Nutritional intervention for women with gestational diabetes should be designed to achieve normal glucose levels, while maintaining appropriate nutrition and weight gain. Many obstetrical centers insist on nutritional counseling, with caloric intakes targeting 30 calories/kilogram of pre-pregnancy body weight per day for non-obese women. As examples, for a woman of average height weighing 70 kilograms (154 pounds) before pregnancy, this would mean a daily intake of 2,100 calories, whereas a woman weighing 60 kilograms (132 pounds) would be advised to eat about 1,800 calories per day. For overweight women (BMI of 30 or more), a dietary target of 25 calories/kilogram of pre-pregnancy weight is considered optimal. As an example, a woman weighing 100 kilograms (220 pounds) prior to pregnancy would be advised to eat about 2,500 calories/day once pregnant. Too few calories over an extended period of time can induce ketosis, which causes profound harm to the developing fetus. No specific ratios of carbohydrates, proteins, and fats have been well studied, but avoidance of excess high glycemic carbohydrates and saturated fats seems prudent. There is no known benefit for eating "funny" fats—i.e., partially hydrogenated vegetable oils—and they should also be avoided. An individualized exercise program incorporating daily walking, swimming, and/or stretching for thirty to sixty minutes appears safe and effective for most pregnant women and may help maintain control of metabolism and glucose levels.

Many obstetrics and high-risk centers have resources to teach their diabetic patients about finger-stick glucose testing at regular intervals throughout the day. Recommended targets for glucose control in gestational diabetics are: fasting levels less than 95 mg/dL; one hour post-meal (also called postprandial) values less than 130 to 140 mg/dL; and two hour post-meal levels below 120 mg/dL. Insulin therapy may be recommended if glucose levels are repeatedly above the target values, and this is done at the discretion of the doctors in charge.

Doctors commonly use a special blood test called the hemoglobin-
a1c to monitor how well their diabetic patients are controlling blood
sugar levels.

Although some women are in denial about their diabetes, failure
to test or report accurate numbers to their health providers only increases the risk to the fetus. Babies of diabetic mothers are much
more prone to birth defects, unusually large size (called *macrosomia*),
and even death *in utero* stillbirth. Before the full significance of gestational diabetes was appreciated, older studies pointed to very high
perinatal death rates in undiagnosed or untreated women.

The ongoing health and well-being of the fetus is usually assessed
in gestational diabetics by several key indicators: First, there is a weekly
or twice-weekly analysis of the fetal heart rate over a twenty to thirty
minute period by attaching a fetal heart monitor to the mother's abdomen (called a nonstress test). A second type of analysis of fetal
movements and amniotic fluid quantity around the fetus is carried
out by ultrasound (called a biophysical profile). Serial ultrasound exams at weekly intervals can determine interval growth and provide an
estimate of fetal weight. The goal with careful fetal assessment in
women with gestational diabetes is to maximize chances for delivery
of a healthy, full-term baby. Good glucose control in the mother correlates well with reduced risks for a complicated delivery or neonatal
period. Additional problems, such as preterm labor or hypertension,
can certainly complicate the prognosis, but most obstetricians and
maternal-fetal medicine specialists are experts in this arena. For high-
risk pregnant women who live in geographic areas far away from such
specialists, consultation and hospitalization (when necessary) has been
shown to improve the outcome for both mother and baby.

BABIES LARGE AND SMALL

It is not surprising that the growth characteristics of babies *in utero* are
highly dependent on the health and metabolic state of the mother.
The fetus derives its macronutrients (carbohydrates, amino acids, and

fats) and micronutrients (essential vitamins and minerals) from the mother's bloodstream. These substances course through the mother's arteries to the uterus and placental implantation site, where placental villi soak and float like water plants within the nutrient-rich lakes of the intervillous circulation. The blood in the intervillous spaces is 100 percent maternally derived, and the trophoblasts lining the villi work to absorb and filter vital substances. When doctors speak of drugs, hormones, or even infectious agents that "cross the placenta," they are referring to the trophoblast layer lining the villi that provides the first defense. Within the core of each rootlike villus are fetal blood vessels—arteries and veins—that both receive maternally derived substances and deliver fetal waste products back to the mother.

By twelve weeks of pregnancy, a fetus weighing just a few ounces has developed fully formed organs and tissues, including bone, muscle, and fat. Once early embryonic development during the first trimester is complete, the fetus becomes capable of dramatic growth. An overnourished mother will often produce an overnourished fetus, and gestational diabetes heightens the risk for having an extra-large child at birth. When glucose levels are elevated in the diabetic mother, excess carbohydrate calories "cross the placenta" to the baby's circulation. The baby effectively becomes overnourished *in utero,* and the fetal pancreas responds by producing too much insulin. This is an interesting situation in which insulin overproduction precedes insulin resistance, since there is no reason for fetal tissues to be resistant to insulin action. Insulin, along with other members of the insulin hormone family, such as IGF-1, stimulates excessive tissue growth and fat deposition.

Extra-large Babies

Macrosomia (from the Latin for "large body") has traditionally been defined as an infant weighing more than 4.0 kilograms at birth, or about 8 pounds, 13 ounces. For many years babies weighing more than 8 pounds were in the upper 10 percent of weight according to gestational age. By today's standards in the United States, that doesn't

really seem so large, and many practitioners now consider macrosomia to be significant for babies weighing more than 4.5 kilograms, or
about 10 pounds. Overnourishment before and/or during pregnancy
dramatically increases the risk of macrosomia. Very obese women
have an eightfold higher chance of delivering a baby that weighs
more than 10 pounds. One in five women who are undiagnosed or
not treated for gestational diabetes will deliver a macrosomic baby.

The greatest risk to the baby with macrosomia is a horrible obstetrical complication called *shoulder dystocia*. In this life-threatening
emergency, the baby's head is delivered vaginally but one shoulder
becomes stuck behind the mother's pubic bone. Various maneuvers
can be attempted to free the baby's shoulder, but this can result in
prolonged injury and nerve damage to the baby, as well as a lack of
oxygen. The risk of shoulder dystocia is highest in babies weighing
more than 10 pounds (4.5 kilograms) born to nondiabetic mothers,
and 8 pounds 13 ounces (4.0 kilograms) for diabetics. Many obstetricians prefer elective cesarean delivery to avoid the risk of shoulder
dystocia, although one study estimated that more than 400 extra cesarean sections would have to be performed to avoid one case of
shoulder dystocia. Ultrasound is often used to estimate the fetal
weight prior to delivery, but a precise measurement is not usually possible. According to a recent ACOG Practice Bulletin, "Planned cesarean delivery to prevent shoulder dystocia may be considered for
suspected fetal macrosomia with estimated fetal weights exceeding
5,000 g (11 pounds) in women without diabetes and 4,500 g (10
pounds) in women with diabetes." A general trend toward higher
birth weights in the United States has contributed substantially to the
rate of cesarean deliveries, which now hovers around 25 percent. Despite this fact, elective induction of labor is not widely advocated as a
preventative measure, creating a significant dilemma for the nation's
obstetricians.

Stunted Growth

About 10 percent of babies are considered small for gestational age, typically weighing less than 2.5 kilograms (5 pounds, 8 ounces) at birth. While *in utero,* a fetus below the tenth percentile in size as determined by ultrasound is considered to have intrauterine growth retardation (IUGR). Maternal factors account for most cases of IUGR, with hypertension and diabetes as common underlying medical problems. IUGR often occurs concomitantly with gestational hypertension and preeclampsia, because blood flow through the uterus and placenta is restricted. Other factors, such as preexisting maternal vascular disease, clotting problems, and the presence of antiphospholipid antibodies (described in the last chapter) can worsen the risk for IUGR. Fetuses exposed to teratogens, cigarette by-products, and infections may have stunted growth and other problems *in utero.* Genetically abnormal fetuses are often growth-retarded and genetic testing is sometimes recommended. Although many small babies are healthy and do well after delivery, consultation and monitoring by high-risk specialists is prudent when IUGR is diagnosed, since underlying maternal problems may be discovered and treated.

A WORD ABOUT OUR NATION'S "LABOR" FORCE

Every year about 1,100 graduating medical students opt for a career in women's health, with a four-year residency in obstetrics and gynecology the most common postgraduate pathway for additional training. During that time, residents work an average of sixty to eighty hours a week in the hospital, caring for some of the highest-risk and sickest patients. When entering practice as specialists in obstetrics and gynecology, these doctors have already logged more than 12,000 hours in direct patient care. Some newly minted obstetrician/gynecologists may choose two to three more years of fellowship training, allowing them to practice as subspecialists in reproductive endocrinology, maternal-fetal medicine, gynecologic oncology, or urogynecology.

The Society for Maternal Fetal Medicine has about 1,600 members who are board-certified or eligible in both obstetrics/gynecology and maternal-fetal medicine. They provide twenty-four-hour consultation and availability around the United States, along with the nation's 25,000 practicing obstetricians. Countless other nurses, nurse midwives, anesthesiologists, and neonatal specialists work around the clock to provide incredible care to our nation's pregnant women and newborn children. In any twenty-four-hour period, about 11,000 babies are born in the United States, and this devoted labor force is available to handle any unpredictable complexity that modern childbearing can create.

All over the country, a real crisis is emerging in women's health, affecting primarily the specialty of obstetrics care. Many experienced obstetrician/gynecologists are closing their doors to new patients or are limiting their practice to just gynecology. Others are retiring earlier than they had planned. To make matters worse, fewer graduating U.S. medical students are choosing specialty training in obstetrics and gynecology. Although numerous factors are to blame, including soaring medical malpractice rates and cuts in health insurance reimbursements, ACOG has issued a "red alert" to the public at large. Access to quality care for pregnant women is seriously threatened.

It is more important than ever that traditional values of positive thinking, creativity, and willpower prevail to solve this crisis in health care. At a personal level, there are responsible changes you can probably make to lessen the health risks to yourself and your future children. Many of the high-risk pregnancy problems outlined in this chapter are preventable, particularly with effective and practical-minded education and motivation. As such, a reduction in overnourishment and insulin overproduction prior to pregnancy appears to be a very worthwhile goal.

BIRTHING HEALTHY BABIES: KEY MOTIVATIONAL POINTS

Tina's story teaches us that there can be many hidden pregnancy pit-falls associated with Syndrome O, including preterm labor and delivery, high blood pressure during pregnancy, and diabetes. Her victorious outcome the second time around also reminds us that old-fashioned attributes like positive attitude, determination, and hard work can make all the difference in the world. Some key concepts to consider:

- Preterm labor and delivery is a scourge on many societies, both in the United States and throughout the world. Currently, about one in eight babies are born before the thirty-seventh completed week of pregnancy. Although modern neonatal medicine helps the majority of preterm babies, many others succumb to severe disabilities or death.
- Although not acknowledged years ago, overnourishment and obesity contribute substantially to the risk of premature labor and delivery. Other factors, such as diabetes, hypertension, and vascular disease are also contributory, but the specific impact of insulin overproduction to preterm birth appears likely.
- Reduction of preterm birth risk may best be accomplished by tackling obesity and overnourishment prior to pregnancy, particularly if encouraged by reproductive endocrinologists and other women's health providers. Current medical techniques to predict or reduce preterm births once pregnancy has occurred have not been particularly effective. Preterm birth in the United States costs about $11 billion per year.
- Hypertensive disorders can impact as many as one in five pregnancies. Preeclampsia is a whole-body disorder that can rapidly threaten the health of mother and baby. Abnormalities associated with preeclampsia mirror many tissue and organ effects of Syndrome O. There is growing concern that

insulin resistance and insulin overproduction contribute substantially to the risk and severity of pregnancy-related hypertension.

- Gestational diabetes affects 2 to 5 percent of all pregnancies,
  but the risk is growing in relation to growing rates of maternal obesity and less-than-optimal preconception health. Syndrome O women should be tested for diabetes prior to
  fertility care, and prevention strategies prior to pregnancy
  should prove beneficial. Pregnancies affected by gestational
  diabetes need extra monitoring of mother and baby.

- Fetal growth can be directly affected by preexisting medical
  problems in the mother, including diabetes, hypertension,
  vascular disease, and pro-coagulant tendencies. Extra large
  babies (macrosomia) can suffer life-threatening problems at
  delivery. Extra-small babies (intrauterine growth retardation)
  may lack life-giving nutrition for proper organ development.

- The professional workforce committed to healthy pregnancies number in the tens of thousands in the United States,
  and many are on-call twenty-four hours per day to handle
  every conceivable pregnancy-related emergency. Society needs
  to value the work of these dedicated individuals.

EIGHT

THE INSULIN BUSTERS:
NEW HOPE OR HYPE?

PALEOLITHIC NOSTALGIA

Food was an obsession for our ancestors. Anthropologists have learned that early humans of the Paleolithic era spent all of their time hunting, fishing, gathering food, and making tools, clothes, and shelter. Despite frequent famines and other acts of nature, the fittest survived through the ages by a combination of inherited and creative talents. Hormonal signals connecting the metabolic and reproductive systems were needed for survival. Even today, the DNA and genes controlling those signals haven't changed much since that time.

In order to understand mankind's modern metabolic needs, it is interesting to consider the nutritional challenges and rewards available to our ancestors of that era. As "hunters and gatherers," a pattern was established of burning calories while looking for food to supply new calories. Protein was a central necessity for maintaining strength and endurance during the quests for food. In the idyllic days of Paleolithic man, protein-rich foods were everywhere—on the land, in the sea, and even in the sky. Of course, we really don't know exactly how much protein humans consumed in that era. Fast food meant that hunted animals moved quickly to avoid being caught! Gathered fruits and berries provided an occasional carbohydrate treat, and essential fats were found in abundance in some organs of the wild prey, as well as in eggs and fish. The meat itself was quite low in fat content. One might ponder: How did Paleolithic humans possibly survive without 50 percent or more carbohydrate calories in their diet, as recommended by our government's Food Pyramid?

Some nutritional experts and anthropologists argue that human advancement really only occurred in the Neolithic era, a time when mankind gradually learned to grow and harvest grains, rice, and other plant products. With this new knowledge, the ravages of famine and harsh weather were offset by longer-term growth and storage of carbohydrates, making survival achievable for many more humans. Agriculture-based societies thrived and grew throughout the world, replacing or co-existing with the Paleolithic hunters and gatherers. Human metabolism reflects both traditions, since most of us are neither purely *carnivore* (flesh-eating) nor *herbivore* (plant-eating). In the course of evolution, human enzymes and hormone systems developed the incredible capacity to utilize calories obtained from plants and animals simultaneously, making us *omnivores* (i.e., able to eat just about anything at any time). Paleolithic humans survived on high-protein diets in the absence of abundant carbohydrates because of enzymes that converted amino acids to glucose. Neolithic and modern humans have survived with less protein because agriculture required less rigor and caloric burn than hunting and gathering. Furthermore, agriculture-based societies also learned how to domesticate and breed livestock and fowl for reliable sources of meat, eggs, and milk.

Most cultures around the world, particularly in the past few hundred years, adopted a balance between the Paleolithic tradition of hunting and gathering and the Neolithic modes of agriculture and animal raising. Some cultures have prospered with more vegetables and starches relative to protein, while other societies thrived with higher protein diets relative to carbohydrates. Subtle nuances in the actions of metabolic enzymes led to tremendous diversity in nutritional requirements among the world's peoples. Yet until recently, most of the world's population was lean and fit.

Thousands of years from now, how will anthropologists view our culture? Mankind's current preoccupation with convenience and food abundance might label our time in history as the "Lazylithic era," or perhaps the "Sedentarylithic era." Future scientists will be in awe of how large empires of food, chemical, and drug companies kept mankind temporarily content for a few hours at a time with processed nuggets of salted and preserved animal flesh, wheat, sugar, and fake fats. When our genes and enzymes clearly couldn't handle the over-abundance, drugs kept us alive and happy, so our people could continue to grow wider, if not taller. Is there a better way to maintain the human condition for future generations?

Due to tremendous diversity in the world's population, it is un-likely that one specific dietary plan can or should apply to everyone. The following are my ideas about how to achieve a healthier, more fertile nutrition plan.

FOOD FIGHT: A SMORGASBORD OF INFORMATION

Unfortunately, the answers about food choices are not cut-and-dry. In order to design an ideal and individualized nutritional plan, it is necessary to consider your options. Many other authors are eager to tell you exactly how you should eat. Have they ever met you? Do they know what foods you like or dislike? Have they examined you, or measured one solitary hormone level or blood test? Do they know your family history? Are they aware of your occupation, and what ac-tivity level it requires? Do they know your age, sex, or ethnic back-ground? Are they clear on your motivation for improving your health and whether pregnancy might be on the horizon?

Obviously, the answer to all of these questions is a resounding "No!" Rather than laying out another diet plan (which can also be found in 28,000 other books), it is more useful to provide you with educated opinions and guidelines, based on scientific knowledge of enzyme pathways and the experiences of Syndrome O women. I've read many of the same diet books that you've read and have identified some pros and cons to each approach.

The fertility and pregnancy risks of obesity and overnourishment are very real. *Your* approach to proper nutrition requires *organization* and planning, *optimization* of *your* food purchases and eating habits, and a desire to *offer your* new knowledge, support, and time to others. Despite only three macronutrient calorie sources to choose from—protein, carbohydrate, and fat—many humans seem faced with an infinite range of poor food choices.

Many psychologists believe that eating patterns and emotional satisfaction linked to food start in childhood and that both genetics and environment play distinct roles. Since most people in our society are no longer required to hunt or harvest, a major information gap has emerged. Neither children nor adults are well educated about healthy food options. The average supermarket is fully stocked with fresh food items; much of it is from farms, slaughterhouses, and waterways. Yet thousands more items are processed, preserved, and stored in cans, jars, plastic containers, and boxes. The challenges facing overnourished people are monumental, yet no one is forcing anybody to eat unhealthy foods in excess quantities. Despite various tempting choices and easy food availability, there are really just three broad types of dietary approaches to consider. Each has its pros and cons for women with Syndrome O.

Dissecting the P-diets

The P-diets refer to the immensely popular, yet often criticized, high-protein diets. Such diets draw upon Paleolithic nostalgia to tell us how we should eat in the modern era. On the surface they make some sense, since our Paleolithic ancestors were primarily carnivores who roamed the planet for thousands of years. In the process, humans developed an efficient enzyme system for converting protein and fat calories to glucose. Biochemists refer to this process as *gluconeogenesis* (i.e., new production of glucose). Enzyme pathways of gluconeogenesis also allow the body to use its own fat and protein as fuel when little or no food is available. Proponents of the P-diets believe that when few carbohydrates are consumed, the body will draw on stored fat by activating enzymes of lipolysis and gluconeogenesis. This is accomplished by keeping insulin levels low, thus slowing the creation of new fats. One biochemical marker in the body to prove that fat is being burned is the creation of little hydrocarbon molecules called *ketone bodies*. The chemical cleaner acetone is a ketone molecule, and people who are actively burning fats may release odoriferous ketones like acetone in their breath and urine. This process is called ketosis. Although mild and temporary ketosis is easily reversible, the impact of ketosis on the ovaries, follicles, and developing eggs is unknown. During pregnancy, ketosis is strongly discouraged.

Although some physicians, such as the late Dr. Robert Atkins, have promoted P-diets for many years, general doubt and negativity have pervaded the medical and nutritional sciences community. Some have labeled P-diets as unsafe and unproven, particularly for people who already suffer or are at risk for heart disease, diabetes, high blood pressure, and high lipid levels. Many nutritionists argue that even if modern man was meant to eat like the Paleolithic humans, we don't know what diseases would have afflicted ancient humans if their life expectancy extended beyond twenty or thirty years. Another cogent point is that animal meat during Paleolithic times was very different in content from today's common meat sources, which often contain high amounts of saturated fat, hormones, and antibiotics. Paleolithic animals, including humans, were active and lean and lived off the land. Most animals that are now bred for human food are underactive and fat. They are fed an overabundance of grains to achieve exaggerated weights and better flavor for the human palate. The long-term healthfulness of P-diets could also be questioned when excessively high quantities of processed meats (containing nitrites, abundant salt, and other chemicals) are eaten.

In the short run, just about any diet plan will produce weight loss if it is carried out as part of a well-monitored research protocol. However, a 2002 published study carried out at Duke University received a great deal of attention by closely evaluating the impact of a P-diet on fifty-one overweight study subjects. The lead author was Dr. Eric Westman, and the results were published in the *American Journal of Medicine*. Although fifty-one people were initially enrolled, forty-one participated and completed the entire six months of monitoring and evaluation. Study participants were placed on a very low carbohydrate diet (less than 25 grams, equal to 100 calories of carbohydrates per day) but without any calorie restriction of protein or fat. They were also given vitamin supplements, information about exercise, and were required to attend group sessions at the research clinic.

After six months, the Duke researchers found some positive results for the 80 percent of original participants who completed the study. Weight loss occurred for most participants and averaged about 10 percent of original body weight, with a range of 5 to 15 percent. Body fat decreased by an average of 3 percent, although some individuals may have lost protein mass as well. Cholesterol and triglyceride levels improved significantly for most participants, and no adverse reactions were reported among the people who completed the study. The researchers concluded that "a very low carbohydrate diet program led to sustained weight loss during a six-month period," and that further research is needed. Although some would debate whether beneficial results after six months predicts sustained weight loss beyond that time, the initial metabolic impact of the P-diet in this study was quite favorable.

However, P-diets may not be for everyone. On a longer-term basis it has not been determined that P-diets have any advantage over other approaches. Once enzymes of gluconeogenesis are turned on by a lack of carbohydrates in the diet, amino acids (the building blocks of protein) act as readily available substitutes. The initial insulin-lowering effects of P-diets may easily become blunted as the body converts amino acids to glucose fuel. Dietary fats are also utilized as fuel, and without attention to overall caloric intake, overnourishment can quickly take over. My experience has been that many Syndrome O women have tried P-diets with moderate initial success, but eventually reach plateaus. The highly restrictive nature of P-diets regarding carbohydrates leads to cheating, and sometimes compulsive over-eating of previously denied foods. Once lipogenic enzymes return to full activity in the presence of excess carbohydrates, the vicious cycle of overnourishment starts again.

Canvassing the C-diets

Excess fat has been blamed for many health problems related to overnourishment, and for years it seemed straightforward to assume that people were eating too much fat. Animal fat was considered the chief culprit, particularly in the form of saturated fats. According to proponents of C-diets, the ideal way to eliminate obesity and cure metabolic diseases like heart disease and diabetes is to eliminate fat al-most completely from the diet and increase carbohydrates. In the ab-sence of dietary fat, overnourished individuals can use their enzymes of lipolysis to gradually break down fats throughout the body, espe-cially in clogged arteries that threaten blood flow to the heart, brain, and limbs. C-diets are usually based around abundant choices of fruits, vegetables, soy and tofu, and whole grains, although varying quantities of low-fat dairy, yolk-free eggs, and limited amounts of fish and seafood may be permitted. Vitamin and mineral supplements are often advocated, and more recently, newer knowledge about es-sential dietary fats has also emerged. Supplements of omega-3 fats like fish oil and flaxseed oil are often recommended in some of the newer modified C-diet approaches.

Does research support the value of C-diets? More than twenty years ago, the late Dr. Nathan Pritikin published six different articles about study results and opinions regarding C-diets. In a group of non-insulin-dependent diabetics, his group demonstrated significant long-term improvements in metabolic indices such as fasting glucose and lipid levels. The Pritikin approach advocates abundant high-fiber fruits, vegetables, and whole grains, and complete avoidance of foods con-taining fat and processed high glycemic carbohydrates. It is completely opposite to the P-diet. C-diets usually include a plea for increased exercise, which helps significantly with carbohydrate caloric burn.

Dr. Dean Ornish has carried the recent banner for low-fat nutrition as the foundation for reversing heart disease. He has published several articles and books that call for generalized life-management change as the way to widen already constricted coronary arteries. An article in the well-respected journal *Lancet* in 1990 noted that: "Comprehensive lifestyle changes may be able to bring about regression of even severe coronary atherosclerosis after only 1 year, without use of lipid-lowering drugs." In that study, twenty-three of twenty-eight patients showed regression of stenosis in their coronary arteries. In a followup analysis in 1998 published in the *Journal of the American Medical Association,* Dr. Ornish and eleven other coauthors found that: "More regression of coronary atherosclerosis occurred after 5 years than after 1 year in the experimental group. In contrast, in the control group, coronary atherosclerosis continued to progress and more than twice as many cardiac events occurred."

In addition to low-fat nutrition and exercise, other lifestyle changes that improved overall health included stress reduction through meditation and yoga, smoking cessation, frequent group psychological support, and leave of absence or retirement from high-stress jobs. Although potentially lifesaving and life enhancing to the individuals involved in his studies, Dr. Ornish's holistic approach may not be completely practical for many people functioning in the real world.

More recently, an interesting article by Dr. J. W. Anderson and colleagues at the University of Kentucky appeared in a 2000 issue of the *Journal of the American College of Nutrition.* Using computer modeling, Dr. Anderson's group evaluated the long-term health benefit of eight different popular diet plans, ranging from P-diets to C-diets. Their endpoint was the potential for coronary heart disease, based on popular recommendations of both caloric and fat intake. Although their study did not involve real people, the conclusion was that "higher carbohydrate, higher fiber, lower fat diets would have the greatest effect in decreasing serum cholesterol concentrations and, thus, the risk for coronary heart disease. While high fat diets may promote short-term weight loss, the potential hazards for worsening risk for progression of atherosclerosis or atherosclerotic events override the short-term benefits."

What can be learned about C-diets as they relate to women challenged by Syndrome O? In my opinion, there are no apparent health risks to C-diets, although like P-diets, their impact on fertility and pregnancy has never been evaluated. However, an important recent study published in 2003 by Dr. P. G. Crosignani and colleagues in Milan, Italy, provides an important link between modest weight loss and restoration of ovulation and fertility. Their article, published in the highly regarded journal *Human Reproduction,* showed that spontaneous ovulation can often occur with just 5 percent weight loss. This was comparable, if not superior, to results achieved in other studies with insulin-lowering drugs, such as metformin. Ten percent weight loss, if achievable, was even more apt to restore fertility in this study. The average BMI of the study participants was 32 (corresponding to a weight of 180 pounds in a five foot three woman). No fancy medical treatments were prescribed, other than a 1,200 calorie per day diet, with daily calorie percentages of 55 percent carbohydrate, 20 percent protein, and 25 percent fats, along with 30 grams of fiber. Essentially this is a C-diet. Aerobic exercise, such as swimming or dancing, was advised at least once or twice per week. Overall, 60 percent of the women ovulated spontaneously and 40 percent became pregnant within twelve months of enrolling. None of these women used or required fertility medications!

The restrictive nature of C-diets may result in cravings, and there is ongoing uncertainty about which lipids are necessary for good health and fertility. The so-called "bad" LDL cholesterol is completely eliminated in the C-diets, even though LDL cholesterol is an essential nutrient for steroid hormone production. LDL cholesterol is absolutely required for production of progesterone, androgens, and estrogen in the ovaries, as well as steroid hormones that are produced by the adrenal gland.

C-diets and P-diets, though seemingly at opposite ends of the nutritional spectrum, have two important features in common. First, they both advocate a complete elimination of foods containing trans or "funny," fats—i.e., partially hydrogenated vegetable oils, or *trans* fats. Secondly, all processed foods containing high glycemic carbohydrates are avoided. There is no way to predict how any individual will react or feel while utilizing a C-diet or P-diet. For many, a moderate nutritional and life-management plan that utilizes insulin-lowering foods from both C- and P-diets may provide an optimal longer term strategy.

Omnivores and M-diets

The history and evolution of mankind's metabolic enzymes demonstrates that we don't really need to be restrictive in our choices of *healthy* foods. However, just as prehistoric man learned to avoid poisonous mushrooms and berries, modern humans should learn to be selective about food quantity and quality. Everyone has food preferences and dislikes, and there are some foods that create allergies and other health problems. Obviously, no specific food should be forced on anyone.

Nutritional plans that advocate moderate portions of high-quality carbohydrates, proteins, and fats seem to make a lot of sense. That is a big disappointment to many overnourished people looking for easy answers. Doctors and other health professionals can clearly identify individuals who are overweight, but it is virtually impossible to know exactly how the problem occurred. Weight gain happens gradually for most people, even those who are overweight. By example, if an individual is overnourished by 100 calories per day—the equivalent of less than one regular soda a day—that person will typically gain about twelve pounds in a year. Being overnourished by as little as 25 calories a day will lead to thirty pounds of weight gain after ten years! Overnourishment can be eliminated immediately by increasing activity and exercise relative to the number of calories eaten. There is nothing fancy or fad about that.

Proponents of P- and C-diets are probably both correct when they proclaim that excess carbohydrates *and* fats contribute to metabolic disease. As discussed in chapter 3, insulin production by the beta cells of the pancreas is disrupted by both excess glucose and fatty acids. Furthermore, not a single expert in the fields of metabolism and nutrition has proposed any health benefit or minimum daily requirement of trans fats.

So what is the true culprit? My guess is that our diet is often comprised of too many high glycemic carbohydrates, many of which contain trans fats. These funny fats are found in many high-sugar foods, such as cakes, crackers, pudding, icings, and cookies, since they add flavor, moisture, and texture. Elimination of these foods from an overnourished diet may provide a double benefit. Since funny fats were first discovered in 1911, humans haven't evolved any new enzymes to metabolize these substances. There is increasing concern that trans fats gradually become incorporated into cell membranes and other fatty portions of our bodies, thus interrupting the flow of many critical hormones' signals. Insulin, along with other insulin-related hormones, relies 100 percent on the vitality of cell membranes to carry out proper metabolic functions.

Many M-diets spell out an exact percentage of proteins, carbohydrates, and fat calories that should be eaten. One popular ratio is 30:40:30 of proteins:carbohydrates:fat. Ratios do not imply anything about quantity. One can be 30:40:30 eating 1,500 calories or 4,500 calories per day. There is no reliable scientific data to support any exact percentage of macronutrients in the diet, although 30:40:30 may be a good moderate starting point for many overnourished people. For a prior way of eating that may have been 10:30:60 in an overnourished individual, 30:40:30 could provide a much healthier ratio. P-diets are commonly skewed to 30:10:60 (the Duke study utilized as little as 5 percent carbohydrate calories), whereas C-diets might have ratios of 20:70:10 (with 10 percent fat as the maximum permitted by Dr. Ornish).

M-diets that advocate 30:40:30 moderation are sometimes incorrectly referred to as high-protein diets. While it is true that they advocate higher protein intake than C-diets, they also tend to admonish the unrestricted saturated fats permitted in P-diets. Dr. Barry Sears is a well-known proponent of an M-diet called The Zone, and he has written numerous books surrounding that theme. He is noted for several different witticisms like: "Eat the way your grandmother told you to eat," and "Treat food like a drug." As a lipid biochemist, Dr. Sears believes that insulin-lowering nutrition plans must include generous portions of low-glycemic fruits and vegetables and proteins that are low in saturated fat (such as poultry and seafood) but higher in omega-3 fats. Since it may be difficult to purchase foods that are high in omega-3 fats, Dr. Sears advocates fish oil supplements. Many scientists are looking closely at the significance of omega-3 fats with regard to a multitude of disease prevention, but the verdict is not yet in.

Some critics consider M-diets like The Zone simplistic and restrictive, particularly for individuals who are very overweight. Yet, other M-diets are strongly advocated by organizations such as the American Heart Association and the American Diabetes Association. The public generally finds M-diets boring and hard to maintain, probably because they do not promise an obvious quick fix. Physicians and dieticians recommend them because they are sanctioned by large official nonprofit organizations. In 2003, the South Beach Diet, created by cardiologist Dr. Arthur Agatston, became a popular M-diet. The philosophy behind this plan is described as neither low-carb nor low-fat. Instead, it focuses on the quantity and quality of carbohydrates eaten each day. The preference is toward natural carbohydrates (primarily fruits and vegetables) that allow for gradual absorption of sugar into the bloodstream—carbs with a low glycemic index. One major difference from other M-diets is that the South Beach Diet doesn't restrict or count calories. This sounds appealing, as long as activity levels and exercise match or exceed daily caloric intake. Otherwise, overnourishment will readily return.

Nutrition and physiology experts in academic and government circles understand that since weight is usually gained slowly, weight loss cannot be expected to occur rapidly. Efficient and thrifty metabolism, with preservation of excess calories, is the norm for mankind. Health professionals who care for overweight people everyday know that weight regulation involves a complex intertwining of more than just metabolism, but also emotions, stress, self-esteem, relationships, and motivation. While food choices are an important element of the overnourishment epidemic, each individual must find some important truths within their own heart, mind, and soul.

WHAT SHOULD SYNDROME O WOMEN EAT?

Every Syndrome O woman needs an individualized personal nutrition plan, but not necessarily a diet. Until biochemical or genetic tests exist to test each person's metabolic enzyme profile, it is simply not possible to tell you what combinations of foods will "work" for you. It is not reasonable to expect any one physician, author, or other professional to know how your metabolism is functioning at any given time. Nevertheless, there are a plethora of ideas to work from, many of which may make sense for your specific goals. Here are some guidelines to consider:

1. *Calories in = calories out.* Although this simple equation seems antiquated, it dates back to the days of Isaac Newton and applies to any machine or organism. You can immediately put a halt to overnourishment by adjusting the quantity and timing of calories you eat, relative to the quantity and timing of calories you burn. Eating a lot of calories late in the day and before going to sleep is one example of how poor timing leads to overnourishment. The appropriate quantity of carbohydrates in your diet may vary from day to day depending on your activity and exercise levels.

2. *Water is your friend.* Staying hydrated allows metabolic enzymes to work at peak efficiency. Water also helps flush out by-products of metabolism. It is easy to become dehydrated, but hard to drink excess water. Excessive thirst and urination can be a sign of diabetes and should be evaluated.

3. *Sugar water is not your friend.* Many women drink large quantities of soda and fruit juices throughout the day, sending

insulin levels into the stratosphere. Overnourishment can often be diminished dramatically by cutting out these empty, difficult-to-burn calories. For a nice fizz, try a calorie-free inexpensive favorite—seltzer water—or its chic cousin, naturally carbonated mineral water.

4. *Diets don't burn calories, activity does.* There is no diet in the world that will substitute for exercise and activity. While it is true that insulin-lowering diets may reverse lipogenic activity in the liver, fat calories still need to be burned in order to eliminate them from the body. The body will burn calories while in motion or at rest, and ongoing exercise improves efficiency of caloric burn, even at rest.

5. *Eat early and often.* Three or more meals per day may actually help to keep your insulin levels within a narrow range. Many uninformed Syndrome O women do not eat breakfast, which starts their metabolic enzymes on a confused path for the entire day. In many instances, Syndrome O women have extremely high early morning insulin, suggesting that too many calories were eaten the previous evening. This may reduce hunger in the morning, but eventually the body catches up and overcompensates. The ovaries do not appreciate high insulin levels at any time of the day or night.

6. *No one is forcing you to eat.* You are the only person who really controls what goes in your mouth. Despite careful planning, if you cannot control food cravings or frequent episodes of binge eating, you could probably benefit from counseling. One good place to start for appropriate professional and support resources is your local chapter of Overeaters Anonymous.

7. *Experiment with food, but not with pills.* While certain prescription medications exist to help with weight loss, only a physician who is willing to evaluate you regularly should prescribe them. Long-term risks of weight-loss medications are not known and should be used with caution. Do not borrow another person's weight-loss remedy. Any non-FDA

approved, over-the-counter pill or herbal supplement claiming weight-loss miracles should be completely avoided. They may be very unsafe.

8. *Try the 5 percent rule.* Most of my patients are comfortable striving to lose 5 percent of their current body weight. Although it may take a few months to lose 5 percent, it will provide tremendous benefit to the vicious cycle of overnourishment and insulin overproduction. Exercise is usually required and is highly recommended for improving insulin sensitivity. Try being undernourished by an average of 250 calories per day, which is readily achievable by most people. If that is accomplished consistently for six months, Newton's laws would predict a fifteen-pound weight loss with any sensible diet. Twenty minutes on a treadmill burns about 100 to 150 calories, and there are many other physical activities that can be enjoyed, particularly outdoors. Many of my patients are eager to lose another 5 percent, which can pose more of a challenge, but should certainly be encouraged.

9. *Eating some fat won't make you fat.* But eating the wrong fats, like trans fats, *will* make you fat. Aim for healthy, lower-fat cuts of fresh meat and poultry, eat eggs and high-fat dairy products in moderation, and strive for omega-3-rich foods like ocean-grown fish and seafood. It is hard to endorse high amounts of additional omega-3 fat supplements until more research is carried out. However, 2 to 4 grams per day of supplemental purified cod liver oil and/or flaxseed oil will probably not cause any harm. Multivitamins with folic acid help lipid metabolism and are a must. Use neutral fats for cooking, like olive and canola oil, and eat dry-roasted, unsalted nuts in moderation. Avoid fries, chips, rinds, and anything cooked with shortening, lard, or partially hydrogenated vegetable oils.

10. *Push away from the table.* Many diet plans do not squarely address the issue of satiety because it is a complex biochemical process in the brain. Scientists are constantly learning new

information about the interaction between food and hormones, but until we learn what truly makes people satisfied, we may not solve the overnourishment epidemic. Psychologists believe that problems such as unhappiness, unresolved interpersonal conflicts, an unfulfilled desire to achieve, guilt about underachievement, and jealousy all contribute to the "never satisfied" syndrome. If issues such as these are holding you back from eating properly and thinking clearly, please seek help from a qualified professional. Use food only as a fuel, and as an occasional supplement to a happy social event or celebration.

A ROLE FOR GASTRIC BYPASS OR BANDING SURGERY?

Many overweight women and men have given up depending on diets, and have turned to gastric surgery to help with long-term weight loss. This may be a reasonable course of action for very obese women desiring fertility and pregnancy. However, a significant degree of life-management change and motivation is required following surgery. Reputable surgeons who perform gastric bypass or banding operations (usually via laparoscopy) usually insist that their patients undergo extensive counseling both before and after the procedure. There is a paucity of published studies evaluating fertility or pregnancy outcomes in women who have had gastric surgery. The information currently available is reassuring. I personally cared for a woman with Syndrome O who underwent IVF one year following laparoscopic gastric banding. As of this writing, she is doing well in her pregnancy.

Take a Hike

The old-fashioned yet essential work of finding and preparing food required significant energy expenditure. There were no alternatives. The communal spirit of ancient tribes and cultures meant that all able-bodied individuals—men and women—were expected to work hard for the betterment of the group. Although strong work ethics and pursuit of nutrition still pervade much of our instincts and thought, the type of work required has changed. Automation and convenience have robbed millions of people of the opportunity to burn calories throughout the day and to maintain metabolic stability.

Placing blame on modern society for inactivity and subsequent disease is interesting from a sociologic perspective, but accomplishes little for those who really need more physical activity. The simple statement coined by Nike rings true for everyone with metabolic dysfunction: "Just do it."

Walking is one of the best ways to get back into a routine of physical exercise after years of inactivity. Unless you are injured or disabled by a problem affecting your body or limbs, there really aren't any good excuses for not exercising. Fortunately, most of us were born with two healthy legs and the ability to walk many miles. There is nothing new to learn. A simple one-mile walk can burn 100 calories or more. Most Syndrome O women can easily increase their walking pace and distance well above one mile once they establish a routine. Very quickly, a chronic pattern of overnourishment can be halted in its tracks.

Some women complain that they experience very little additional weight loss after a few weeks of sensible eating and exercising. Part of the explanation lies in the fact that exercise increases muscle mass while fat tissue is gradually reduced. This contributes to increased muscle-related weight, which can add slightly to overall body weight. But don't despair! Improvement in muscle function is the key to eliminating insulin resistance. As the muscles become more capable of utilizing glucose efficiently, less glucose is available for conversion to fat. Likewise, insulin overproduction stops. For Syndrome O women, this is essential to sparing the reproductive system from the harmful effects of excess insulin. A healthy diet of low-glycemic carbohydrates, moderate proteins, and the right fats will work together perfectly with your new exercise routine.

Exercise and Syndrome O

Scientific journal articles regarding the benefits of exercise for Syndrome O, along with a sensible M-diet, are gradually appearing. Dr. Robert Norman, who leads a reproductive medicine unit at the University of Adelaide in Queensland, Australia, has been a strong proponent of lifestyle management. His group has published data in several articles that demonstrate a dramatic improvement in insulin sensitivity and reproductive function after six months of balanced eating and exercise. Weight loss was modest, in the 2 to 5 percent range of original body weight, suggesting that muscle mass was added. With improved metabolic indicators, a number of women participating in Dr. Norman's studies achieved spontaneous ovulation and a few became pregnant.

It is not feasible for me to spell out the details of your individualized exercise routine. I've never met you, and I don't know your body size, health history, or daily schedule. Although walking is a great way to get started, there are many other combinations of aerobic and anaerobic exercise that could help you improve insulin sensitivity. Exercise has also been credited with reducing stress and poor sleep patterns through better functioning of the adrenal gland. There are many resources available to women who truly want to take control of their metabolism and stress levels through exercise. One excellent book that is worth a look is called *Real Fitness for Real Women: A Unique Workout Program for the Plus-size Woman*. It was written by Rochelle Rice, a respected certified fitness instructor in New York City. Her approach utilizes proper low-impact aerobics and strength training with a greater focus on physical activity rather than diet. Ms. Rice has also demonstrated a particular interest in helping infertile women with Syndrome O achieve maximal metabolic balance.

Although most Syndrome O women have experienced challenges with weight during much of their lives, about 10 to 20 percent of Syndrome O women are not overweight and may actually be quite thin. Although insulin resistance *per se* may not be a contributing problem, I do believe that thin Syndrome O women are also overnourished. Although their absolute insulin levels may be in the normal range based on standard lab criteria, it is likely that their sensitive ovaries are still confused because of imbalances in the insulin family of hormones. A diet of excess carbohydrates, coupled with inactivity and low muscle mass, can easily cause Syndrome O in a thinner woman. For such women, attention to carbohydrate intake and exercise can also greatly improve glucose utilization, leading to lower insulin levels. Essentially all women with Syndrome O can benefit from improved muscular function and tone, along with moderate increases in muscle mass.

DRUG PEDDLING: YEA OR NAY?

Many Syndrome O women go to their doctors expecting a magic pill or remedy. Although the metabolic challenges faced by Syndrome O women are often quite significant, the opportunity for life management change *without* the use of drugs is vast. Seeking help from a knowledgeable physician is a terrific first step, but if you've read this far it should be obvious to you that Syndrome O is not curable with one simple pill. Society's preoccupation with convenience often leads people to assume that doctors can prescribe pills for just about any ailment. Some doctors' preoccupation with time constraints and overwhelming office responsibilities leads them to hand out pills without a lot of patient education or hands-on evaluation. We are lucky to have an armamentarium of good medicines to treat people affected by a variety of diseases. However, overcoming Syndrome O also requires personal responsibility and life management, in partnership with appropriate and conservative medical care.

Soon after the Nobel Prize–winning discovery of insulin in the 1920s, some endocrinologists, such as Dr. William Wolf, suspected that ovarian function was particularly dependent on insulin action. He wrote in the 1936 textbook *Endocrinology in Modern Practice:* "The islands of Langerhans [containing the insulin-producing beta cells of the pancreas] have been credited with having a definite influence upon the ovarian secretions." In women who lacked insulin, due to what would now be termed type 1 diabetes, "the administration of insulin resulted in the cure of their sterility." Dr. Wolf also pointed to evidence in animal studies that "administration of insulin reduces fertility due to the fact that it inhibits ovulation." The conclusion in the 1930s by certain endocrinologists was that ovulation and ovarian function are dependent on specific quantities of insulin.

The clinical significance of insulin *overproduction* on the ovaries was not appreciated in 1935 when Drs. Irving Stein and Michael Leventhal first presented and published findings from seven women with polycystic ovaries and a lack of menstrual periods. For years, Stein-Leventhal syndrome, also called polycystic ovary syndrome, was believed to be a primary disease of the ovaries, best treated by removing large portions of ovarian tissue. For almost fifty years after the first description of Stein-Leventhal syndrome, the link to metabolism and insulin overproduction eluded gynecologists and most other physicians. Clomiphene, surgical ovarian wedge resection, and gonadotropins became the mainstay of therapy in the 1960s for this relatively uncommon infertility condition.

Physician scientists, such as Dr. Robert Barbieri and the late Dr. Ken Ryan at Harvard University in the early 1980s, are widely credited with establishing a significant link between insulin resistance and androgen overproduction in the ovaries. They proposed that insulin resistance resulted in compensatory insulin overproduction, leading to two key aspects of Syndrome O—ovarian confusion and ovulation disruption. In a landmark study in 1984 published in the journal *Ob-*

stetrics and Gynecology, their lab found that insulin and LH worked synergistically to stimulate androgen production in the stromal connective tissue and theca cells of human ovaries.

Metformin (Glucophage), a drug that is FDA-approved for treatment of type 2 diabetes, has been studied for many years, with more than two thousand journal articles, dating back to the 1960s, catalogued in the National Library of Medicine. It has several mechanisms of action that allow the body to utilize glucose more efficiently, thus reducing insulin overproduction. Despite the profound increase in cases of Stein-Leventhal/polycystic ovary disorders seen through the 1980s and '90s, the potential value of metformin wasn't readily obvious to most doctors. Nor were many health professionals making the connection to nonmedical treatments like nutrition and exercise.

Dr. E. Valazquez and colleagues at the University of the Andes in Merida, Venezuela, reported the first use of metformin as medical treatment for polycystic ovaries in the journal *Metabolism* in 1994. Many of their study patients experienced significant reductions in blood insulin and androgen levels after eight weeks of taking metformin at a dose of 1,500 mg/day and some had ovulatory menses and pregnancy without using fertility drugs.

In 1996, Drs. John Nestler and D. J. Jakubowicz, at the Medical College of Virginia in Richmond, helped clinch the link between insulin overproduction, androgen overproduction, and the ovaries by publishing a landmark article about metformin in the *New England Journal of Medicine.* They found that metformin dosages of 1,500 mg/day had four important insulin-lowering reproductive and metabolic effects: First, it reduced the activity of an enzyme directly involved in androgen synthesis; second, it reduced insulin levels in response to a glucose challenge; third, it reduced LH levels; and fourth, it directed the liver to increase levels of SHBG—a vital sponge protein that binds to "free" androgens. Overall, metformin created a more favorable insulin and androgen environment allowing follicle growth and ovulation to occur. Drs. Nestler and Jakubowicz confirmed this impression with a followup landmark article in the *New England Journal of Medicine* in 1998.

Since 1994, numerous other research groups have studied the value of metformin for treating the co-existing clinical challenges of insulin resistance, androgen overproduction, and ovulation disruption. As of this writing, 150 journal articles have been cataloged by the National Library of Medicine with the key words "metformin" and "ovary," and 61 have been published with key words "metformin" and "ovulation." Many of these are articles that review the work of others. In one excellent 2003 review about metformin, written by Dr. Barbieri in *Obstetrics and Gynecology,* a total of 21 original scientific articles were identified that met stringent criteria for evaluating the clinical effectiveness of metformin in the following settings important for women: 1) ovulation induction; 2) menstrual cycle irregularity; 3) hirsutism; 4) pregnancy; 5) adolescence and puberty; 6) prevention of diabetes; 7) weight reduction; and 8) prevention of endometrial cancer.

It is important to stress that studies regarding the overall risks and benefits of metformin for Syndrome O women are works-in-progress by the medical and scientific community. The potential value of metformin to all Syndrome O women is so important that the National Institutes of Health is currently devoting millions of dollars to a prospective multicenter study titled: "Randomized Study of Decreased Hyperinsulinemia on the Ovulatory Response to Clomiphene Citrate in Women with Polycystic Ovary Syndrome." At the time of this writing, study subjects are being recruited around the country.

Women who wish to become pregnant and who are willing to be randomized without their knowledge to receive either metformin or placebo, in addition to clomiphene, can join the study. Certain other criteria for study entry include ovulation disruption and/or anovulation, elevated androgen levels in the bloodstream, and a willing male partner with a normal sperm count. For a full description, visit www.nichd.nih.gov/new/releases/ovary_syndrome.cfm.

The following institutions are currently participating in this multicenter study: Penn State Milton S. Hershey Medical Center (where Dr. Richard Legro heads the entire study), along with Baylor College of Medicine in Houston, Hospital of the University of Pennsylvania in Philadelphia, University of Alabama at Birmingham, University of Colorado, University of Medicine and Dentistry of New Jersey at Newark, University of Texas Southwestern Medical Center, Wayne State University in Detroit, University of North Carolina at Chapel Hill, Virginia Commonwealth University, Stanford University, University of California at San Diego, and University of Pittsburgh.

Until we have clearer answers from this large-scale study, which may take a number of years to fully interpret, it is reasonable for doctors to be cautious and conservative in their use of metformin as treatment for Syndrome O. Also, this new NIH trial does not include a study "arm" evaluating sensible nutrition and exercise compared to metformin, nor a study "arm" that includes both. This is unfortunate, since a major publication in 2002 by Dr. Knowler and colleagues in the *New England Journal of Medicine* showed that lifestyle intervention was far superior to metformin in the prevention of type 2 diabetes.

My interpretation and use of the information to date regarding metformin for my patients with Syndrome O is as follows:

Ovulation Induction

Metformin appears to be beneficial for lowering insulin and enhancing follicle growth in many women who previously demonstrated resistance to clomiphene. If response to clomiphene is not known in advance, the use of metformin in combination with clomiphene appears more efficacious than clomiphene alone. Metformin also helps ovarian responsiveness when gonadotropin medications such as pure FSH (Bravelle, Gonal-F, Follistim) are used. It has become common in our practice to promote the following sequence prior to ovulation induction: first, strategic lifestyle change three to six months before ovulation induction (see chapter 9); second, discussion of pros and cons of metformin treatment and initiation with patient consent one to three months before ovulation induction; third, stepwise increase from 500 to 1,500 mg/day of metformin prior to prescribing clomiphene or FSH; and fourth, continuation of metformin into the luteal phase and early pregnancy with patient consent and discussion of risks and benefits. Metformin is tolerated well by most women, al-though gastrointestinal side effects are widely reported. A sensible nu-trition plan aimed at reducing simple sugars and trans fats may alleviate many symptoms. Fatal cases of lactic acidosis, although rare, have been reported.

In Vitro *Fertilization (IVF)*

A blockade of follicle growth is not usually apparent in Syndrome O women undergoing stimulation with higher doses of gonadotropins for IVF. Therefore, it is not yet scientifically established that metformin provides a definitive benefit. The theoretical advantages of insulin and androgen reduction prior to IVF stimulation seem reasonable, but it will require some cleverly controlled studies to evaluate the pros and cons. I have used metformin selectively for some IVF patients.

Pregnancy

Metformin has received a relatively benign pregnancy category B designation by the U.S. Food and Drug Administration, suggesting no known evidence of harm to unborn children. A few published re-ports describe the use of metformin during pregnancy to treat gesta-tional diabetes. As discussed in chapter 6, metformin may reduce miscarriage risk in the first trimester and may ameliorate insulin over-production in later pregnancy. Patients in our practice are presented with currently available information and most are motivated to con-tinue metformin usage during the first trimester. We keep a watchful eye for side effects and poor pregnancy outcomes in all of our fertility-care patients.

Weight Loss

Modest weight reduction is a desired result for most women with Syndrome O, as it improves insulin sensitivity. This is particularly true if regular muscle-enhancing exercise is part of strategic life management. Unlike other diabetes medications, such as insulin, pioglitazone (Actos), and rosiglitazone (Avandia), which tend to increase weight, the impact of metformin on weight is more hopeful. Effects on appetite, gastrointestinal absorption, and lipolysis via enhanced insulin sensitivity may all contribute to modest weight loss while taking metformin. Weight loss is generally not encouraged during pregnancy.

Other Benefits

As will be discussed further in chapter 10, the improved androgen profile brought about by metformin can help with cosmetic issues such as hirsutism, hair thinning, and acne. An improvement in coagulation profiles is evident with metformin, particularly since PAI-1 (discussed in chapter 6) protein levels are reduced. This may reduce risk of thromboembolic events (blood clotting in veins and arteries), and may improve perfusion to coronary arteries, the brain, and the limbs. Diabetes prevention has been clearly demonstrated, but this likely necessitates a combination of both metformin and lifestyle management. Whether or not the effects of metformin and lifestyle are additive has not been scientifically established, but good sense would suggest a combined benefit in the shorter term. The very long-term risks versus benefits of metformin, or any other insulin-sensitizing drug, have not been established for the prevention or treatment of any particular disease or metabolic disorder.

Glitazone Drugs

Current insulin-sensitizing drugs in the thiazolidinedione class, such as pioglitazone (Actos) and rosiglitazone (Avandia) also have potential for treating Syndrome O women. The research thrust and clinical enthusiasm with these medications has been hampered by the market withdrawal in March 2000 of troglitazone (Rezulin) due to fatal incidents of liver toxicity. Many doctors now use glitazone drugs to help overcome insulin overproduction and ovulation disruption, since there are reports that they are better tolerated by the gastrointestinal tract. In some clinics, both metformin and a glitazone drug are pre-scribed together as dual therapies. One newer concern about glita-zone drugs is the direct inhibition they appear to have on ovarian steroid production, independent of their insulin-lowering impact.

COMING OUT OF HIBERNATION:
KEY MOTIVATIONAL POINTS

Key points to consider are:

- Human nutrition has undergone significant transition since our Paleolithic ancestors roamed the earth. Although prehis-toric men and women survived primarily as carnivores—eating mostly protein and not much carbohydrates—the more recent Neolithic era gave mankind agriculture and wider control over food choices. Heredity and metabolic enzymes have given humans the luxury of deriving nutritional benefit from protein, certain fats, and unprocessed carbohydrates.
- Nutritional advice is everywhere, and it is largely based on opinion rather than rigorous scientific studies. Tremendous genetic diversity among the world's population suggests that one specific dietary plan will not apply universally.
- Three general approaches to nutrition currently exist, based on daily quantities and proportions of protein, carbohydrate, and fat. P-diets profess that 90 percent or more of daily calo-ries should be derived from protein and fat in an unrestricted manner. C-diets are quite the opposite, suggesting unlimited and high proportions of grains, fruits, and vegetables in the diet, with less than 10 percent of daily calories from fat. Moderate proportions of macronutrients constitute M-diets.
- Overnourishment can easily be eliminated by limiting caloric intake to the quantity of calories burned through physical ac-tivity and exercise. Chronic overnourishment leads to weight gain by insulin overproduction and enzyme pathways pro-

moting fat production. Being overnourished by 100 calories per day will add twelve pounds of weight in one year.

- Syndrome O women should follow guidelines for healthy nutrition and design their own personal plan for eliminating overnourishment. Exercise is the only way to burn calories that have been stored as fat. A sensible M-diet, utilizing low glycemic index carbohydrates, moderate quantities of protein, and an absence of trans fats will achieve longer-term metabolic control.

- Exercise, even the simple activity of walking, will greatly improve insulin sensitivity in the muscles. As the muscles become conditioned to burn glucose more efficiently, the body's tendency to overproduce insulin and store fat is eliminated. Many resources are available to help overweight women achieve better metabolic control through exercise. Movement is a must, even during pregnancy, when it can be gentler; there is no substitute.

- Drugs to enhance insulin sensitivity, such as metformin, may prove to be important adjuncts for helping Syndrome O women achieve normal reproductive function. Since 1994, studies continue to be carried out demonstrating enhanced ovulation function in response to metformin. Caution and conservative management is prudent until large scale prospective multicenter trials are completed.

- Drugs like metformin are unlikely to be the "magic bullet" for eliminating Syndrome O, or other diverse metabolic diseases such as diabetes, hypertension, heart disease, and health problems associated with insulin overproduction. Responsible life-management strategies will likely achieve more far-reaching and satisfying results.

NINE

SOS: TURNING TO THE SYNDROME O SURVIVAL STRATEGIES

A Few Small Steps Equal One Big Step

Women with Syndrome O are faced with tough challenges everyday, including lifestyle adjustments and real health concerns. Often, they feel overwhelmed and don't know where to turn for help. "I need to be pointed in the right direction" is a common plea. We all feel stressed and inundated with work at different times in our lives, and many of us become inefficient, depressed, and withdrawn when faced with too many tasks and responsibilities.

Despite these pressures, and all the new information from this book that must be absorbed, the following small steps are a necessary starting point. To achieve goals, Syndrome O women must begin by believing in themselves.

- *Don't panic.* Help for Syndrome O can come from a number of excellent sources, including your own strong desire for self-improvement.

- *Start thinking.* Your mind is your strongest ally. Actions and decisions of the past must be kept in perspective while you decide on a plan for the future. Focus on the good things in your life.
- *Begin living.* You have much to offer yourself and others. Experience everything you can, especially in the great outdoors, even if it is in your own backyard.

The Syndrome O Survival (SOS) Strategies provide a blueprint to give Syndrome O women a fighting chance for enhancing their fertility and health. "You will accomplish that which is important to you" is the philosophy that forms the foundation of the SOS Strategies, a framework for living that complements and enhances the necessary medical evaluation and treatment for Syndrome O.

Education, Motivation, Stimulation

Taking steps to improve one's life is courageous and empowering and can only enhance the overall prognosis and help you beat Syndrome O. However, this empowerment can only be achieved through a fully integrated approach. Initially, women must first learn about Syndrome O through *education.* Read and learn everything you can. And never stop asking questions! Finding the *motivation* to change requires deep reflection, meditation, and a willingness to pursue goals and desires. *Stimulation* implies being nudged by yourself and others who care about you to really go after those goals. Stimulation also requires moving up the SOS pyramid to the next stage—to seek and pursue professional medical evaluation and opinion.

The Value of Time

One important premise that allows the Strategies to be successful is the notion that each person universally owns 24 hours per day and 168 hours per week of a very precious resource—*time.* Only you

A Syndrome O Strategic Pyramid

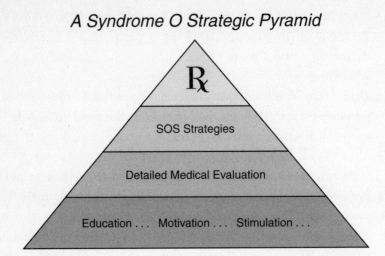

control the time you spend on various activities, and you may believe that you currently don't have enough time to devote to life management and good health. In order to change that notion you may need to modify your belief system about time and start to use it in an *organized* and *optimized* fashion. It will then become possible for you to *offer* time, both to yourself and others, for productive activities that promote health, vitality, and good deeds in your community.

Rediscovering Your Talents

Every Syndrome O woman I have met has at least one *talent,* which can be developed and structured to enhance self-worth and self-esteem. When working to overcome Syndrome O it makes sense to capitalize on every positive aspect of your life. Talents can be small or expansive—like having a kind voice, an artistic flare, a knack for caring about others, or being a terrific cook—and can encompass virtually any aspect of your life. Why waste your talents on negative thinking or self-deprecation? Talents tend to grow and blossom, and they can be put to use in so many worthwhile ways. When you draw on your talents for the betterment of yourself and others, you will naturally find that you are using time more efficiently. Motivated and stimulated people know that time spent on self-realization and expansion of talents is one of the essential ingredients to having a good life.

Personalize Your Treatment

Treatment is defined in different ways and may encompass medications prescribed by a physician, surgical procedures, and professional counseling. Taking excellent care of yourself is also a vital component of Syndrome O treatment, which includes paying closer attention to nutrition, physical activity, stress, and sleep. If fertility and a healthy pregnancy is your major goal, then fertility treatments may necessitate a significant change in your daily routine. In order to *optimize* the effectiveness of your fertility care choices, you will need to *organize* every aspect of that care, including issues of informed consent, anticipating success or disappointment, and the very real financial costs. The more time and talent you *offer* to your treatments, the more committed you will be. As you demonstrate ongoing devotion to this goal, the interactions that you develop with your doctor and other clinic staff will allow them to offer you the most help possible. Likewise, being patient and fostering avenues for constructive communication will provide you with the best odds for success. Great patients tend to find great doctors, and vice versa.

Putting the SOS Strategies to Work

	Time	Talent	Treatment
ORGANIZE			✓
OPTIMIZE			✓
OFFER			✓

The Three Strategic O's

The SOS Strategies invoke three very important principles—organization, optimization, and offering. This three-pronged approach is balanced, like a strong and stable three-legged stool, and encourages equal devotion to each strategy. With the SOS Strategies, women with Syndrome O can find enhanced healthfulness and happiness in their lives.

A wonderful example of a real person who has been instrumental in putting the principles of SOS Strategies into practice is Lesa Childers. You will read more in chapter 12 about her personal experiences and perspectives with the challenges of Syndrome O, as well as her professional endeavors in social work and counseling. Lesa's energy and dedication to helping others with the SOS Strategies, as well as the nonprofit organization she now leads (www.pcostrategies.org), have inspired many other women to achieve fertility, an ongoing commitment to healthy living, and most important, personal life fulfillment.

I have collaborated with Lesa for over five years as the SOS Strategies have evolved from blueprint to reality, and I asked her once, "Why do you believe it is important for women with Syndrome O to develop an individualized and strategic plan?" Her answer truly helps define the mission of the SOS Strategies:

> One of the beauties of the human existence is our individual uniqueness. Each person experiences life in their own special way according to their physical makeup, environmental influences, and mental/emotional perceptions. While women with Syndrome O exhibit similar physical symptoms to one extent or another, there is no way to prescribe one "cookie cutter" plan that works for everyone.
>
> Each of us is at a different point in our Syndrome O journey, making decisions every day about how to deal with the diverse challenges we face. Developing a personal plan encourages self-examination and prioritization of life goals. As we travel the path of our life goals, priorities

often change, and therefore change the journey. For instance, eight years ago my number one aspiration in life was achieving pregnancy. In order to reach that goal I had to develop a plan that was unique to me and my life circumstances. My strategic plan is different today, as I am in a different place in my life. While others can learn from my personal experiences, the "Lesa Childers plan" was specific only for me.

Women with Syndrome O need much more than just good medical care. They need positive and constructive guidance to create personal strategies that put knowledge into action.

MAKING PLANS: THE SOS STRATEGY OF ORGANIZATION

When life seems to be spinning out of control, it is time to pause for a deep breath and make a commitment to the strategy of organization. Just as there are lots of self-help diet books, there are plenty of experts who are paid to write about how you should organize your life. Frankly, only you have the brainpower and insight to organize your days, weeks, or years. Organizing yourself to overcome Syndrome O may require some deep thought and the *ongoing* willingness and commitment to ask some tough questions of yourself. I don't have the answers, only you do.

Organize Your Goals and Desires

What do you really want to achieve in your life? What are your strengths? What are your talents? What is stopping you from reaching for your goals? How do you envision yourself and your family in one year? In five years? In ten years? Is your career or profession a priority? How does time for family and friends fit in? What is the status of your relationship with your partner or spouse? Is having a child or more children a strong desire? Are good health and quality of life important to you?

Focusing on a single objective can have profound benefits to your entire life plan. Anthony Robbins, who is both an amazing showman and motivational speaker, calls this principle the "concentration of power." He writes in one of his best-selling books, *Awaken the Giant Within:*

> One reason so few of us achieve what we truly want is that we never direct our focus; we never concentrate our power. Most people dabble their way through life, never deciding to master anything in particular. In fact, I believe most people fail in life simply because they major in minor things.

Many women tell me that they have actually been quite happy with their relationships and career choices. Unfortunately, as time passes, they may have allowed their health and family-building aspirations to take a back seat. They may have made erroneous assumptions about the physiology of their reproductive systems, or were told misinformation. One important lesson of the SOS Strategies is to *forgive your past,* and to *focus on the future.* For example, overnourishment habits should automatically change if one is truly committed to reducing insulin overproduction and healing the body in preparation for fertility and pregnancy.

Is dedication to your career and a strong desire to help others actually circumventing your ability to help yourself? Dr. Frank Hu and his colleagues at Harvard Medical School followed 85,000 female nurses from 1980 to 1996, all of whom were considered healthy and free of disease at the beginning of the study. There are few professions that measure up to nursing when highlighting a professional group that is both informed about healthy lifestyles and has a desire to help others. Unfortunately, during the sixteen years of the study (published in 2001 in the *New England Journal of Medicine*), 3,300 new cases of type 2 diabetes were documented within the group, representing 1 out of every 26 nurses. Only 3.4 percent of the 85,000 nurses were considered to be at low risk for diabetes based on personal lifestyle management. The study predicted that many more nurses from this group have become diabetic since 1996 or will develop diabetes in future years. The lesson here was that while nurses are often helping others with significant health problems, they may be ignoring their own health needs. The authors concluded that the majority of nurses in the study were not capitalizing on their education and knowledge about obesity, poor diet, and lack of exercise. They had not created personal action plans for maintaining their own good health.

If you love your job, then love yourself also, and give your health and fertility the priority it deserves. If you dislike your job then consider finding a new one, particularly if a change will help you achieve goals of good health and motherhood. As a compromise, try to identify aspects in your current work that can be improved or modified. Recruit your coworkers, friends, family, and partner or spouse to support your newly organized focus and decisions for positive change.

Organize Your Time

You may now believe that you don't have enough hours in the day for all of life's activities. In order to arrange time for the things that are truly important, you may need to constantly remind yourself about your most important priorities. You must concentrate and control your power over time! Rich or poor, fat or thin, smart or less-than-gifted, we all have the same 168 hours of living to do in any particular week. As part of the strategy of organization it is crucial to be accountable for your own 168-hour week. How many hours do you spend at work? How many hours with family? How many hours at rest? How many hours at chores? How many hours have you committed to overcoming Syndrome O through education, motivation, and stimulation?

In my practice I hear a lot of "I don't have time to _____." You can imagine many different ways to fill in the blank: "eat right," "buy fresh food," "learn how to cook healthy meals," "attend support meetings for watching my weight," "go to the gym," "take a walk," "find out more information about Syndrome O," "take a yoga class," or "take care of myself." Hopefully, you've had time to read this book, and I hope that effort on your part will prove worthwhile.

No one can create more time for you. The clock moves at the same speed for all of us. What you can do for yourself is to closely evaluate the important activities in your life and eliminate those that are unimportant and incompatible with your goals and desires. Watching the evening news on television may be important and worthwhile to keep you informed about world events; settling into the couch for three hours to watch old sitcom reruns, accompanied by 1,000 calories of sugar water and snacks, is probably not very productive (or insulin reducing). Reading about fertility care or weight management on the Internet could be very informative; spending fifteen hours per week in an online chat room is not likely to help you accomplish anything.

Most Syndrome O women are highly productive individuals, striving for excellence in their lives and the betterment of others. Many women are extra tough on themselves, putting achievement ahead of personal contentment. I consider this part of the "never satisfied" syndrome, leading to internal unrest, extra stress, and unexplainable discontent. One hallmark of this phenomenon is a disorganized approach to nutrition and exercise: grabbing bad foods and snacks on the run; missing meals; gorging when voraciously hungry; or sitting for hours into the night working at a computer or talking on the telephone. Poor sleep patterns add additional stress to already overworked adrenal glands and worsen insulin overproduction. Interestingly, women at completely opposite ends of the work and productivity spectrum can often suffer with the same Syndrome O problems.

The choice is therefore yours to make. If you can get organized and find the time to eat properly, exercise regularly, and get appropriate sleep, you can help adjust your insulin overproduction on your own. This is one goal of the SOS strategies: Can you make the commitment?

Organize Your Approach to Health Evaluation and Treatment

Taking steps to strategize one's life is courageous and empowering and can only enhance the effectiveness of your health care. As part of the process, do some careful research and ask some important questions before settling on a particular doctor, clinic, or counselor. Make a list of your Syndrome O symptoms, in the order that bothers you most. Use the twenty-five-question list "Could I Have Syndrome O?" in chapter 1 as your guide. It may not be possible for your physician to help you with every problem at the initial visit, so it could help your doctor tremendously if you are clear on your chief complaint, or better put, *your number one goal.*

In my specialty, the desire for fertility is usually the number one goal of most of my patients. However, there are many other health or cosmetic concerns that are commonly associated with Syndrome O and may need to be addressed, including desire for weight loss, avoiding the risk of diabetes, or irregular and/or heavy menstrual cycles. Others are worried about depression, anxiety, poor self-esteem, relationships, and career indecision.

Once you have organized your symptoms, you can begin to seek help from the right health-care providers. A fertility specialist who is primarily known for directing a high volume IVF facility may not have much expertise in helping you with more conservative ovulation induction treatments. Doctors who are experts in weight management and exercise physiology may not offer fertility care. Read and learn everything you can, but be very open to expert consultation and opinion. Come to doctor and nurse visits armed with questions, but make sure you are requesting information that is specifically relevant to your care. Be prepared to arrange your life schedule to accommodate both evaluation and treatment phases. If you make an appointment you must plan to keep it, unless a real emergency prevents you from doing so.

As health providers with lives of their own, doctors and counselors can only be expected to devote their precious time to clients who truly respect and desire their help. The more you are willing to organize and commit to helping yourself, the more you will gain from your interactions with dedicated professionals. Not every visit can be expected to proceed flawlessly. There are ups and downs to every doctor-patient relationship. However, with regularly scheduled visits, you should be experiencing steady improvement in knowledge, health, and faith in yourself.

It is wise to hold your doctors accountable for their advice and treatments, even though there are no guarantees in any realm of medicine, especially fertility care. However, consider holding yourself equally accountable for all personal actions that can impinge on your life goals and desires. "The woman is an active participant in her own care," states Dr. Sam Thatcher and Lesa Childers, in a book chapter from *PCOS: The Hidden Epidemic.* "Through an open dialog patients learn the medical basics of their problems and about treatment options. Each member of the partnership respects the other's expertise, and the phrase 'I disagree,' from either side is not met with contempt. Trust is essential and paramount and is built from mutual respect. Mutual respect is the key to long-term success."

Women often find it difficult to locate a health-care provider with expert knowledge of their reproductive health problems, especially if they live in more remote, rural areas. When asked to elaborate on this challenge, Lesa stated, "I advise women to become informed consumers and to learn as much as they can while seeking quality care. They must become knowledgeable about local health-care resources and should research doctors, nurses, and counselors who are within reasonable distances from home or work. Getting the care you need may mean a commitment to travel, or even to move outside your present community." Having honest conversations with those who might be affected by your decisions, particularly coworkers and supervisors, is another important aspect of good organization. In the best of situations, fertility treatments can be time consuming and stressful to your work environment. Taking steps to organize and prioritize your time devoted to these efforts is a good strategy to employ.

Getting Real: The SOS Strategy of Optimization

The SOS Strategy of Optimization provides an uplifting, positive opportunity to focus on insulin-busting and life-enhancing techniques. One exciting aspect of the Strategy of Optimization is that it works to shift your attention from organizing and planning to real action and improvement. There is no better feeling in life than putting a plan into motion and watching it unfold successfully. While there are always excuses to be found, the honest truth is that the only person getting in your way is the person you see in the mirror each day. Some days will be better than others, but aim for optimizing each part of *your* day to the fullest.

Optimize Your Life Activities

Be proactive toward the life goals you identified in the strategy of organization. Are you happy at work? Can you optimize your attitude and activities to bring more joy to the job? Are you content at home with yourself and your loved ones? Can you optimize your home life to bring greater joy to yourself and your family? Can you optimize your relationships with other friends and family?

Every interaction you have with another person can either be *helpful* or *hurtful*. Helpful exchanges create harmony in your body as well as in others. This leads to lower stress and production of happy chemicals in the brain, called endorphins. Scientists have found that *satiety*—contentment with body and soul—is directly related to levels and quantities of these opiate-like natural hormones in the brain. Did you ever notice that some people just seem happy all of the time? Does it necessarily relate to their job, wealth, or station in life?

I often wonder why many people in the services industry—health care in particular—appear so unhappy. You can often see the hurt in their faces. There is the receptionist at the doctor's office that won't look up and greet someone with a smile. There are nurses and doctors and hospital staff who are always angry with patients and with each other. Everyone is entitled to have a bad day, but for many people this becomes a chronic pattern of behavior and discontent with the world.

Are you one of those people who are always angry at the world? Are you frequently hurtful toward those who value your care, knowledge, and expertise? If this is your *modus operandi* in life, then it must stop immediately. Leading a hurtful and disrespectful life toward others will only worsen your inner strife and metabolic well-being. No one can make you become a happier person, but there are numerous resources you can draw upon to help you think and act more positively toward others.

Many people are happy on the outside but sad on the inside. They are kind and give magnanimously in time and effort to others, but are miserable with themselves. This type of disharmony also worsens stress, sleep patterns, and normal metabolic function. Such behavior may indicate organic and life-threatening depression, requiring immediate professional care. Fortunately, it is treatable, both with non-pharmacologic techniques and medications. Clinical depression is a popular disease for the pharmaceutical industry to capitalize upon. Milder cases of the blues don't necessarily require medication. No one can force you to find the resources that might help, but your quality of life could suffer in the meantime. Seeking out activities that truly make you happy—reading a good book, watching a sunset, walking along a beach or lake, writing a letter to an old friend, taking a Sunday afternoon drive—might make you smile more on the inside and release some extra brain endorphins.

Optimize Your Nutrition

Make personalized lists of the foods you like and dislike and decide on priority foods for yourself that are Syndrome O–healthy. Proper nutrition is not really that complicated once you make it part of your routine. Plan ahead to eat a balance of higher protein, smarter fat, and lower carbohydrate M-diet foods on a regular basis. These include leaner cuts of fresh meat, poultry, and seafood, abundant fruits and vegetables, and whole-grain, high-fiber carbohydrates. Decide on quantity and timing of each meal. Avoid eating excess calories late in the day or evening.

Consider joining an established nutrition program like Weight Watchers that meets in your community (there may be other programs that are equally reputable). The cost of such programs is often a factor for many people, particularly when they seek individualized care with certain outstanding dieticians and nutritionists in private practice settings. Some academic and university-based medical centers have nutritional lifestyle programs that are less expensive, but may require you to participate in a research study. By whichever route you take, if you closely analyze the money you might be spending each week on fast foods, junk foods, sugar water, and excess foods, an optimized weekly budget might allow you to spend funds on weight-management and fitness programs.

There is a wealth of resources in books, magazines, and on the Internet, all containing valuable information so that you can become educated, motivated, and stimulated to make the right food choices. Some nutritional gurus push the concept that only naturally grown foods should be eaten. In the past, all foods were natural. Perhaps the healthiest meat sources for us now should come from animals that are not inbred or given high-carbohydrate grains as feed. Leaner meats such as venison, buffalo, and ostrich are gaining popularity, as are fish and seafood that are fresh out of the sea (rather than farm raised). There is evidence that fruits and vegetables grown without pesticides and chemical fertilizers could be healthier. Although more expensive and often inconvenient to obtain, it is possible that our future health would really benefit by eating more natural foods on a consistent basis.

Dr. Andrew Weil is a leading author and advocate of optimizing nutrition naturally. In one of his books, *Eating Well for Optimum Health,* he writes: "When I use the words eating well, I mean using food not only to influence health and well-being but to satisfy the senses, providing pleasure and comfort. In addition to supplying the basic needs of the body for calories and nutrients, an optimum diet should also reduce risks of disease and fortify the body's defenses and intrinsic mechanisms of healing. I believe that how we eat is an important determinant of how we feel and how we age. I also believe that food can function as medicine to influence a variety of common ailments."

When you eat to excess, or eat the wrong kinds of foods (fatty or high in simple carbohydrates) do you really feel satisfied? Ironically, many scientists believe that the consumption of fat is actually the most important component of food that leads to the feeling of satiety. One hormone, leptin, is produced by fat tissue and regulates "satisfaction circuits" in the brain. Some scientists believe that diets higher in fat and protein tend to be more appetite-suppressing. Others promote strict vegetarian diets. What is agreed upon is the fact that different combinations of fats, proteins, and carbohydrates affect our hormones in different ways.

If humans were the same as laboratory rats, we might have more useful scientific answers regarding food and satiety. However, most of us are cultural and ethnic hybrids, with combinations of metabolic genes derived from the far corners of the planet. This metabolic and genetic diversity allows us to enjoy all kinds of foods, sometimes to excess. Therefore, to overcome overnourishment, each of us must experiment with different combinations and quantities of healthy foods to find those that provide the most satisfaction and optimal fuel.

Positive interactions and socialization during meals are helpful and will likely maximize chances for satiety at mealtime. In many families, mealtimes are disjointed or disorganized. Try to rearrange schedules so that meals can be shared in a more relaxed and friendly setting. The fun of eating will be enhanced if it is shared with others.

Optimize Your Fitness

With an organized 168 hours of each week, you should be able to identify at least five hours that you can devote to physical activity. If you cannot find a minimum of five hours each week then perhaps you are working too hard. Otherwise, what is your excuse? It is not fair to ignore people with special circumstances, such as those who are physically disabled or those who are caring for a very ill spouse or family member. Nevertheless, I rarely see Syndrome O women in my practice who have such valid predicaments.

Make lists of the physical activities you enjoy now or did enjoy in the past—walking, bicycling, swimming, dancing, gardening—and do any of the activities on your list for at least five hours each week. It is not necessary to join a gym, although many women have found facilities such as Curves to be very beneficial. Being physically active will help to eliminate overnourishment *immediately*. Burning 400 extra calories five times a week is equivalent to eliminating a full day's worth of food. That will greatly shift the "calories in = calories out" equation in your favor.

Walking at a moderate pace for five to ten hours per week provides women with significant protection from life-threatening cardiovascular events. According to an important study by Dr. JoAnn Manson and her colleagues, who published their results in the *New England Journal of Medicine* in 2002, moderately brisk walking provided the same cardiovascular benefits as more vigorous exercise. Their positive findings were significant irrespective of race or ethnic group, age, or body mass index. They concluded that increasing intensity or duration of exercise led to improved lipid levels and insulin sensitivity. Of particular relevance to women with Syndrome O, "Moderate exercise coupled with modification of the diet led to a reduced risk of type 2 diabetes among subjects with impaired glucose tolerance. Moreover, equivalent energy expenditure with moderate or vigorous exercise leads to similar reductions in adipose mass. Finally, physical activity of any intensity has been linked to improvement in emotional well-being."

Creating a walking fitness program might require a little time for planning and some initial minimal costs for the appropriate clothes and foot gear. I witness positive transformations in my patients every day when they commit their time and bodies to optimal physical activity.

Making Life More Meaningful: The SOS Strategy of Offering

The last leg of the SOS Strategies is the *Strategy of Offering*. Finding meaning within your life can be enhanced by offering yourself to others: kindness, concern, a warm greeting, a sincere thank you, or just a considerate "have a nice day." Showing interest in others is infectious; it sends a positive message to every person with whom you interact, creating a chain reaction of kindness. Having an attitude of offering costs you nothing. Plus, you will find that good feelings generated in your heart and soul will reward you with many little bursts of endorphins throughout the day.

Offer Your Attention to Loved Ones (and to Yourself)

Said the Wizard of Oz to the tin man, who thought he needed a heart: "Remember, my sentimental friend, that a heart is not judged by how much you love, but by how much you are loved by others." Do you spend enough quality time with family or friends? Could this time be spent in a more physically active way (for example, taking a hike)? Could quality time be spent in a more nutritionally healthful way? Do you spend enough time attending to yourself? By offering more attention to your own self-improvement, it will become natural to offer compassion to important people in your life.

Walking, talking, and interacting are the essence of human existence. Sitting on a couch or in front of a computer screen is not. Why not round up the troops—either family or friends—and plan a day of adventure? There's a big country out there, and probably new things to see and do within a short distance of your home. Virtually any activity that gets you moving and interacting with people will result in pleasurable feelings. Reacquaint yourself with younger members of your family network. Your life experiences should allow you to provide some valuable mentoring to kids and young adults. One conversation with a young person may direct that individual toward a beneficial and fulfilling life decision.

Offer Your Time and Expertise Outside the Home

There is a whole community filled with important needs outside of your home and work. Could you offer any special service? Are you active in your house of worship? Is there a particular charity for which you could volunteer? Does your local school need tutors? Does the local school board need committee members? Is there an upcoming political campaign that interests you?

Those who participate fully in their communities view their place in the world very differently. As stated by Paul Rogat Loeb in his 1999 book *Soul of a Citizen,* those who get involved know "that they don't need to wait for the perfect circumstances, the perfect cause, or the perfect level of knowledge to take a stand; that they can proceed step by step, so that they don't get overwhelmed before they start. They savor the journey of engagement and draw strength from its challenges." I believe that there is also a happy medium to this endeavor. Some people constantly offer themselves to others but pay little attention to their own needs. Yet there are others who are self-centered and uncaring. Where do you see yourself in this regard, now and in the future?

The health value to those who offer time as community volunteers has been studied from a scientific perspective. In a study published in 2001 in the *Journal of Health and Social Behavior* by Drs. Peggy Thoits and L. Hewitt at Vanderbilt University, aspects of personal well-being were evaluated in people who worked as volunteers. Over time, their results showed that volunteer work enhanced six important aspects of personal well-being: happiness, life satisfaction, self-esteem, sense of control over life, physical health, and depression. As you develop an organized and optimized philosophy with your time and talents, it is only natural and *healthy* to offer your expertise to those who could benefit.

Offer Your Assistance to the Syndrome O Community

A crucial aspect to successful SOS Strategies is to teach others about the personal approaches that have been helpful to you. No one woman will follow the same path to success with the SOS Strategies. But through local community support groups focusing on nutrition, weight management, and fitness, you will find that your ability to live well and thrive will be enhanced each and every day.

PCOStrategies is a nonprofit organization founded on the premise that millions of women in the United States and around the world could benefit from individual proactive strategies to overcome over-nourishment, infertility, and less-than-perfect health. Thus far, women from throughout the United States have contributed and participated in the mission of PCOStrategies, leading to self-improvements in health and fertility. The notion of give and take is important to the ongoing success of the organization. It is a work in progress, but is likely to form the foundation of how Syndrome O women everywhere can focus their energy to improve their lives.

Ongoing research by PCOStrategies led to the development of a novel online survey to assess the needs and knowledge base of women with Syndrome O. The 635 responses to the PCOStrategies Web site were analyzed over a two-month period and the results were presented at the 2003 national meeting of the American Society for Reproductive Medicine. The authors of the study were Lesa Childers, Dr. Barbara McGuirk (my colleague at Reproductive Associates of Delaware), and myself. Salient findings were:

- 94 percent had been told by a physician that they had polycystic ovaries.
- 80 percent were between the ages of nineteen and thirty-four.
- 46 percent were actively seeking pregnancy.
- 80 percent were concerned about their fertility, now or in the future.

- 94 percent were concerned about their weight.
- 97 percent were concerned about their long-term health.
- 83 percent were concerned about cosmetic issues.
- 79 percent were concerned about their mental health.

Of particular interest:

- Only 19 percent were satisfied with the education they received from their health-care provider about polycystic ovaries
  and other aspects of Syndrome O.
- Yet 78 percent believed they would participate in PCO-
  Strategies educational programs, if available in their area.
- 66 percent agreed with partnerships between nonprofit organizations, such as PCOStrategies, and private health-care
  providers to meet the educational needs of women: 30 percent were undecided about this new concept in patient education.

The survey suggests that a significant gap exists in what health
providers are teaching their patients compared to sources of information that women can find on their own. The majority of respondents
felt they would seek out and participate in PCOStrategies programs
designed to educate, motivate, and stimulate.

BE THE VICTOR, NOT THE VICTIM

It is easy to believe that you are a victim of Syndrome O and all the
other problems associated with it. "I have Syndrome O because
_____" is often completed with statements like: "my mother
fed me bad food," "my father's family has bad genes," "I work at a
desk all day," "I don't have time to eat right," "I have a bad metabolism," or even "my last doctor told me the wrong thing." Accepting
your own imperfections and challenges should not be equated with
being a victim of a problem that others imposed upon you.

There are numerous proponents of "learned optimism," a term coined by Dr. Martin Seligman at the University of Pennsylvania. His premise is that negative thoughts can influence your actions and attitudes about yourself. Learning winning ways to lead your life is actually an old concept made famous by Dale Carnegie in the 1930s during an era of bad economic times around the world. Attitude is everything. "If we think happy thoughts, we will be happy," he said. "If we wallow in self-pity, everyone will want to shun us and avoid us." The old truths are still valid: if you think positively about yourself, you will feel in control, and you can create change.

Syndrome O women are now armed with powerful tools to combat a whole-body disorder that could claim victims, but doesn't have to. Put the SOS Strategies to work to make yourself victorious. Follow the pathways of education, motivation, and stimulation that will allow you to partner with the right doctors and pursue the right treatments. Focus on all the good things you can accomplish and contribute to the world around you. The opportunity is yours, and only yours.

Moving in the Right Direction: Key Motivational Points

- Take some small steps toward the bigger step of overcoming Syndrome O. Despite the effects Syndrome O may have on your fertility and health, the best step-by-step advice includes: 1) Don't panic; 2) start thinking; and 3) begin living.
- The Syndrome O Survival (SOS) Strategies provide a blueprint for giving your health, fertility, and life a fighting chance. The SOS Strategies encompass your time, talents, and treatments and provide you with the impetus to establish a personalized framework for organization, optimization, and offering.
- The SOS Strategy of Organization encourages you to prioritize your goals and life plans, your schedule and time, and

your approach to medical evaluation and treatments. It is vital to decide your number one goal, or chief complaint, when visiting a doctor or counselor.

- The SOS Strategy of Optimization should motivate and stimulate you to take action. Numerous opportunities abound for optimizing your life activities, nutrition, and fitness. There are no good excuses for failing to optimize these aspects of your daily existence.

- The SOS Strategy of Offering allows you to make life more fulfilling, by offering your time, talents, and treatment wisdom to others. There are many acts of kindness you can offer others every day. There are no quotas on offering; the positive impact on your health and well-being could be enormous.

- Decide on a positive mental attitude and follow through on a daily basis. No one likes a whiner. The reasons that you have Syndrome O may be multifaceted, but can be overcome. Be a victor, not a victim.

- Acknowledge the ongoing Syndrome O challenges in your life. With self-improvement and compassionate medical care underway, revel in every small victory. Become empowered with the SOS Strategies, and your health and attitude will improve, weight will drop, energy levels will increase, and your reproductive system will be given a break from the bombardment of excess insulin hormones.

TEN

BEAUTY IS MORE THAN SKIN-DEEP: OTHER SYMPTOMS OF SYNDROME O

WHO MAKES THE RULES?

The price of living in a free and capitalistic society is exposure to a barrage of information that constantly tells us what is attractive, intelligent, and available for purchase. We are all at the mercy of powerful entities in business and the commercial media, who inform us constantly about how to look and feel.

Human vanity has deep roots. Traditionally, both sexes of the gentry class have been responsible for equating appearance with wealth and power. Consider the primping, clothing, cosmetics, and wigs of aristocrats—both male and female—that was desired and lauded for centuries throughout the Western world. In the United States and elsewhere, diverse societies and cultures establish norms for appearance that are whimsical and change frequently. In nongentry classes, which have always encompassed most of the world's people, women have commonly accepted more of the burden for beauty and appearance.

Everyone has the right to decide how much time and attention he or she wishes to devote to mind and body. Nevertheless, we are taught at an early age that whether we like it or not, we will often be judged by how we look. Many psychologists and social scientists believe that more young girls are affected by poor body image than boys, which correlates with many societal expectations of women brought on by both sexes. As stated by psychologist Dr. Margo Maine in her book *Body Wars:* "Beauty is a trap door for women."

Women are often confused by signals of feminism and pressure to seek equal opportunity to men, yet many women also have traditional biologic and social visions of finding a mate, reproducing, and raising children. When women find that their bodies don't look or function normally, this often adds to confusion, sadness, lowered self-esteem, and a less-than-optimal quality of life. Experts who study and treat body image problems have not commonly addressed all the underlying hormonal aspects of Syndrome O. In the future, as reproductive endocrinologists and their patients seek out interactions with specialists in the social sciences and gender psychology, an enhanced view of societal norms, strategic self-improvement, and personal responsibility should unfold.

Understanding Hair Growth

Expectations among women for maintaining smooth and beautiful skin, particularly on the face, have caused many Syndrome O women to feel abnormal, diseased, or even freakish. Two common problems that greatly distress women are facial hair and blemishes caused by acne and hair removal. According to Women First HealthCare and the Bristol-Myers Squibb companies, who comarket the facial cream Vaniqa, about 41 million women in the United States have unwanted facial hair. Most Syndrome O women are among the millions who spend countless hours plucking, tweezing, shaving, and waxing to control unwanted hair growth on their face and other parts of their body. Many find they must attend to this problem on a daily basis. Other women spend a great deal of money and time undergoing frequent electrolysis, laser treatments, and visits to dermatologists. These cosmetic challenges are often described as "nightmarish," and are actually considered more unsettling to many Syndrome O women than weight, infertility, and abnormal menstrual cycles.

Hirsutism is the nasty-sounding medical label applied to women who have excessive body hair. But how is "excessive" hair growth actually defined? For many women, this has traditionally been a hazy area based on cultural and personal expectations. A widely used scoring system was established in 1961 by Drs. D. Ferriman and J. D. Gallway for quantifying hair growth on women's bodies. While some women might consider the Ferriman-Gallway score demeaning and embarrassing, especially when under the care of a male physician, it continues to serve an important purpose for medical evaluation, response to treatment, and clinical research studies.

A detailed Ferriman-Gallway score measures hair growth on an increasing-severity scale of 0 to 4 at twelve different regions of the body, including the upper lip, face, chin, jaw and neck, upper back, lower back, arms, thighs, chest, upper abdomen, lower abdomen, and perineum and inner thighs. These are common spots for women to have undesired hair growth, whether mild, moderate, or severe. A combined score of 8 or greater (out of a maximum of 48) medically defines hirsutism. By that stringent standard, a vast number of women, with or without Syndrome O, would be considered hirsute. Numerous cosmetics, pharmaceutical, and medical industries are eager to capitalize on women's frustration with hirsutism.

Gynecologists and other physicians are trained to be on the lookout for relatively uncommon but life-threatening *virilization* symptoms in women who have shown increased hair growth. Virilization is defined as a rapidly progressing hormonal abnormality leading to dramatic malelike changes, such as growth of a full beard, balding, deepening of the voice, enlargement of the clitoris, and muscular enlargement throughout the body. Androgen-producing tumors of the ovaries or adrenal gland are usually responsible for virilization and can often be malignant. The chronicity and severity of masculinizing symptoms require careful documentation with the Ferriman-Gallway score in order to make a diagnosis and decide on treatment. Fortunately hirsutism, unlike virilization, does not usually point to an emergent or life-threatening medical condition.

THE ROOT OF THE HAIR PROBLEM

Many women are told by their doctors that hirsutism is caused primarily by excess androgens in the bloodstream. This view is simplistic and doesn't take into account many other aspects of metabolic function and the body's glandular internet we have previously discussed. Syndrome O women come to realize that they must often focus on two types of follicles—those that house and incubate eggs in the ovaries, and the tiny structures embedded in the skin that support hair growth. Like the follicles in the ovaries, women (and men) are born with a fixed number of hair follicles.

Heredity determines many features about the body's hair follicles: number, density, and function, along with the quality and color of hair formed by each follicle. The responsiveness of hair follicles to hormones such as testosterone is predetermined by both genetics and the enzymes that process testosterone within the follicles. In all hair follicles, the active androgen is dihydrotestosterone (DHT), which is derived directly from testosterone through the action of one enzyme.

In both men and women, "free" androgens and their conversion to DHT can contribute to *either* hair growth or hair loss, depending on location. Both men and women have frequent consternations about their scalp hair and follicles. Paradoxically, DHT can induce hair loss on the scalp, yet promote unwanted hair growth elsewhere on the body. Unfortunately, excess free androgens and DHT can cause many scalp follicles to permanently cease hair growth. Many Syndrome O women have this problem.

Since the first description of Stein-Leventhal syndrome and polycystic ovaries, an association between hirsutism and excess ovarian androgen production has been observed. In 1990, a group of experts convened at the National Institutes of Health with the mission of

creating a consensus definition to the medical community for polycystic ovary syndrome, or PCOS. Only two definite criteria were
agreed on: hyperandrogenism (i.e., androgen excess) and menstrual
irregularity. Insulin resistance, and even polycystic ovaries were only
considered "probable criteria." (Imagine the confusion generated
amongst doctors and patients when the NIH declared that polycystic
ovaries were not considered a definite criteria for PCOS!) More recent studies with insulin-lowering drugs have supported the notion
that overnourishment and insulin overproduction are the real culprits
linking metabolism to excess androgen production. Definitive proof
came when it was shown that metformin and glitazone medications
can result in substantial reduction of total and free androgen blood
levels.

Excess androgens may not always result in hirsutism. Likewise,
women with hirsutism often don't have elevated blood levels of androgens. Shrewd clinicians understand that *organ sensitivity* to hormonal signals, as in hair and ovarian follicles, largely determines
normal or abnormal function. Many Syndrome O women experience minimal or mild hirsutism initially, but find that the problem
worsens as time goes by. In most cases this can be correlated with the
worsening impact throughout their bodies of overnourishment, insulin overproduction, and ovarian confusion.

The quantity of free, or unbound, androgens is more likely to be
elevated in Syndrome O women than the total androgen level, which
can often be in the normal range. Free testosterone can be measured,
along with levels of a liver sponge protein called sex hormone binding globulin (SHBG). Low levels of SHBG are almost always found
in Syndrome O women and directly correlate with higher levels of
free testosterone. The liver is the body's metabolic "brain" and consequently affects hair follicle activity. As insulin levels increase, the
liver produces even less SHBG, and hair follicles become bombarded
with increasing amounts of free testosterone.

In order to best create a profile regarding androgen production for
each of my patients, I request that certain blood tests be carried out.
As described above, total testosterone, free testosterone, and SHBG

levels in the blood provide good information about the impact of insulin overproduction on androgen production and how those androgens might be affecting hair follicles. To be thorough, I recommend two other androgen-related tests: 1) DHEAS, which indicates how active the adrenal glands (the stress organs) may be in adding androgens to the bloodstream; and 2) 17-hydroxyprogesterone, a marker of an inherited adrenal enzyme deficiency discussed later in this chapter. These tests are important before deciding on the best treatment options.

Thousands of hair follicles throughout the body are potentially subject to ongoing free androgen stimulation, creating ongoing and persistent Syndrome O challenges. Previously dormant hair follicles are often stimulated by excess free androgens, leading to new hair growth throughout the body, including certain predictable areas on the upper lip, chin, face, jaw, and neck. The inherited sensitivity, location, and density of hair follicles primarily determine where and when hair will grow. It is generally believed that once a hair follicle

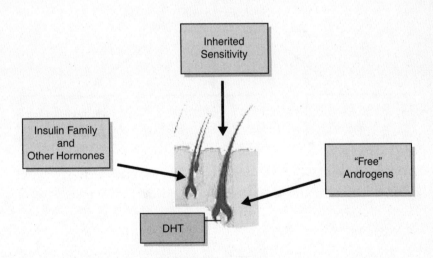

Inherited sensitivity of the hair follicle determines growth of hair in response to "free" androgens and other hormones, such as the insulin family. Within the root of the hair follicle (the dermal papilla), enzymes process and convert "free" androgens to dihydrotestosterone (DHT), which directly stimulates hair growth. On the scalp, excess DHT can promote hair thinning and balding.

becomes newly activated, it has the capacity to produce a hair for years. This is an important concept for the treatment of hirsutism, since each follicle that produces an undesired hair can be treated by an array of temporary or permanent approaches, which will be discussed below.

Overnourishment and obesity present complex and increasingly common challenges to children and teenagers, during a time in their lives when personal identity and self-esteem are crucial to future well-being. Although Syndrome O problems of ovarian confusion and ovulation disruption may occur any time during a woman's reproductive life, a worsening pattern of undesired hair growth may start at a young age and predate reproductive concerns. Symptoms of excess free androgen action—both unwanted hair growth and acne—can start in childhood and adolescence and may be an important early sign of Syndrome O. Studies have shown that insulin also directly af-

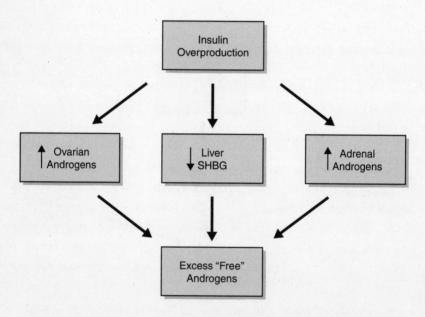

Insulin overproduction is directly responsible for decreased production of sex hormone binding globulin (SHBG) by the liver. Decreased SHBG is directly responsible for increases in "free" circulating androgens, along with increased production of androgens from the ovaries and adrenal glands.

fects enzymes of the adrenal gland, leading to stimulation and production of adrenal androgens. Symptoms of early or precocious puberty in girls can reflect a combined effect of insulin overstimulation of pituitary gland, ovaries, adrenal glands, and the liver. Androgens from the adrenal glands initiate growth of "sexual" hair (armpits, chest, and pubic area) and changes in sebaceous (oily) glands in both girls and boys months before the gonads become activated. As puberty progresses, androgens from both adrenals and gonads contribute to the circulating pool of active blood levels.

MEDICINES THAT CAN HELP

There are no immediate cures for unwanted hair growth. Most women develop a pattern of personal cosmetic measures, which include shaving, plucking, or waxing off existing hair. Syndrome O women commonly carry out these activities on a daily basis.

Medications prescribed by doctors to overcome hirsutism act by preventing or reducing growth of *new* hair in follicles not yet activated by free androgens. The effectiveness of these medications will depend on length of use and androgen sensitivity of the hair follicles. Unfortunately, no medications for controlling hirsutism are considered compatible with the desire for immediate fertility care and pregnancy since they could harm a developing fetus. Many Syndrome O women are requested to stop taking medications that had been used to combat hirsutism and acne several months prior to fertility care.

Although there is no direct proof that life-management changes such as the SOS Strategies will reduce or prevent hirsutism, insulin-lowering strategies will significantly reduce free androgen blood levels. Insulin reduction leads to two important benefits: the enhanced production of SHBG by the liver; and reductions in ovarian and adrenal androgen production. Many researchers also believe that the insulin family of hormones, including insulin and IGF-I, may directly influence the function of hair follicles and sebaceous glands. Within the hair-producing cells of the follicle, DHT and the insulin family work together to stimulate hair growth. In the sebaceous gland adjacent to the follicle, these same hormones act to increase oily secretions (sebum), affecting risk for acne.

As with all medical approaches for management of unwanted hair growth, concomitant insulin-reducing strategies are also likely to be beneficial. Proper nutrition, exercise, stress reduction, and a commitment to restful sleep may all contribute to reductions in free androgens and insulin, leading to longer-term improvements in hirsutism and acne.

Benefits of Birth Control Pills (BCPs)

BCPs were not developed for the control of androgen excess, hirsutism, or acne, but they are now widely prescribed for these problems. BCPs work as effective contraceptives by inhibiting ovulation and preventing the production of pituitary gonadotropins. BCPs break the cycle of androgen overproduction in the ovaries by dramatically lowering luteinizing hormone (LH). Women with Syndrome O tend to overproduce LH, which works with insulin to stimulate ovarian androgen production in the stromal and theca cells. Lower LH correlates directly with lower ovarian androgen production.

BCPs are comprised of combinations of estrogen and progesterone, with an array of doses and formulations available. There is no definite benefit of one brand over another, although physicians should be knowledgeable about the pros and cons of each BCP they prescribe. By virtue of the estrogen component, all combination BCPs will induce the liver to produce greater quantities of SHBG, thus providing additional sponge protein to soak up androgens like testosterone. BCPs are probably the most effective medication available for lowering free androgen levels. Adrenal androgens can continue to swamp the bloodstream, especially when the adrenal glands are under stress. It has been suggested by previous research that BCPs may also provide some mild reduction in adrenal androgens.

In general, BCPs have more benefit than risk for the treatment of hirsutism and acne. However, both the estrogen and progesterone components of BCPs may be associated with a few noteworthy problems. As BCP estrogen stimulates the liver to produce more SHBG, the liver may also respond by synthesizing extra blood clotting proteins. Excess clotting capacity can contribute to *thrombosis* in the veins or arteries, especially in the setting of insulin overproduction. Progesterone in BCPs can also worsen thrombosis risk, as well as contribute to weight gain and insulin resistance. Smoking and BCPs is a bad combination and is greatly discouraged due to heightened risk of potentially deadly blood clots in the legs and lungs. Any woman with a family risk of thrombosis should be evaluated and tested by a hematologist for underlying inherited thrombophilia before starting BCPs (or anticipating pregnancy). All women taking BCPs, particularly Syndrome O women, should be advised of these small, but very real possibilities.

There are also caveats related to the progesterone component of BCPs. Some of the older BCPs contain progesterone compounds that are considered mildly androgenic, which can theoretically blunt the benefits of the estrogen component. Some newer BCPs do not have this effect. A BCP containing norgestimate (Ortho Tri-Cyclen) has even been approved by the FDA for the treatment of acne.

One newer BCP contains the progesterone agent drospirenone (Yasmin), which has been shown to have anti-androgenic activity within the hair follicle. It has functional and structural similarities to another anti-androgen called spironolactone. Blood levels of potassium could be increased by this BCP, and it may not be recommended in certain clinical situations. Although not available in the United States, BCPs containing the more potent anti-androgen cyproterone are widely used in other countries to treat hirsutism. Based on recent research by Dr. H. Seaman and colleagues from the University of Surrey in the United Kingdom, and published in *Human Reproduction* in 2003, BCPs containing cyproterone contribute to increases in thrombosis in women with hirsutism, acne, or polycystic ovaries. It is likely that for those women, insulin overproduction, cyproterone, and the estrogen component all contributed to excess thrombosis risk.

In addition to thrombosis, other strong contraindications to use of BCPs include vaginal bleeding that is undiagnosed, liver disease, breast cancer, and known history of coronary artery disease. For obvious reasons, if you wish to become pregnant now, then extended use of BCPs may not be suitable for you. However, many fertility specialists incorporate short-term use of BCPs into ovulation induction treatment cycles.

Anti-androgens

Spironolactone (Aldactone) is a diuretic and blood pressure–lowering oral medication that has been used for many years to treat hirsutism. It has biochemical activity that blocks DHT synthesis within hair follicles and may bring about mild decreases in ovarian and adrenal androgen production. The medication is generally considered safe, although it may require many months of use to become effective. Spironolactone will not inactivate hair follicles that are already producing hair. Combination treatment with spironolactone and BCPs is commonly recommended, but BCPs containing drospirenone or cyproterone should probably not be used in conjunction with spironolactone.

Two other anti-androgen oral medications—finasteride (Propecia, Proscar) and flutamide (Eulexin)—are occasionally prescribed to combat hirsutism. These medications are typically prescribed to men to treat prostate cancer, benign prostate enlargement, or balding. In some women with unremitting hair growth, these agents may be more effective than spironolactone. No anti-androgens are approved by the FDA for the treatment of hirsutism, and the FDA warns that neither finasteride nor flutamide should be used by women, especially if considering or attempting pregnancy.

A Prescription Topical Cream that Can Help

Eflornithine HCl 13.9 percent (Vaniqa) is the first topical prescription treatment approved by the FDA for the reduction of unwanted

facial hair in women. It acts by inhibiting an enzyme in the hair follicle that produces substances called polyamines, which are necessary
for hair growth. For the majority of women using Vaniqa, unwanted
hair growth will gradually slow, but hirsutism will not be cured. In a
study cited by the manufacturer, 58 percent of 393 women treated
with Vaniqa for twenty-four weeks showed some improvement, compared to 34 percent of 201 women treated with a placebo cream.
Within the category described as "marked improvement," Vaniqa and
placebo were equally effective for 26 percent of women. Fair-skinned
women achieved more benefit than women of African ancestry. As
stated in the patient information insert written by the manufacturer,
improvement occurs very gradually. Women using Vaniqa shouldn't
become discouraged, since it usually takes four to eight weeks of
treatment to see some improvement. For some women the treatment
takes longer, but if no improvement occurs after six months, then the
drug should be discontinued. In women who noted improvement,
hair growth will return about eight weeks after stopping treatment.

Vaniqa cream is recommended for twice-daily use and should not
be used during pregnancy. Although relatively expensive (one 30-gram
tube costs about $120), the manufacturer notes that "a little Vaniqa
goes a long way." A thin layer of Vaniqa should be massaged into affected areas until absorbed. Once it is dry, other cosmetic products
such as moisturizers can be applied. In the clinical trials prior to FDA
approval, some women experienced minor skin irritation, such as
redness, stinging, burning, tingling, or rash. Only 2 percent of study
subjects discontinued use due to side effects. There is no contraindi-
cation to continuing other androgen-reducing medications, such as
BCPs or spironolactone while using Vaniqa. The manufacturer has a
Web site for women who are interested in more information about
Vaniqa (www.vaniqa.com).

An Alternate Hormonal Approach to BCPs

In some women, BCPs are contraindicated or unsafe. In some
instances of severe hirsutism it may be safer and more effective to

temporarily suppress pituitary LH and ovarian androgen production with once-monthly injectable medications such as Lupron, Zoladex, or a daily nasal spray called Synarel. Since these medications also block estrogen production by the ovaries, menopausal side effects may occur (for example, hot flashes, vaginal dryness, mood swings, irritability, and difficult sleep). Prolonged use of these pituitary blockers places women at higher risk for osteoporosis and reductions in bone mineral density. Many women benefit from "add back" therapy with small doses of estrogen and progesterone, which can alleviate menopausal symptoms and protect bone metabolism. Over a three- to six-month period of time with this approach, dramatic reductions in ovarian androgens can be achieved, along with some improvement in SHBG and free androgens.

Metformin and Glitazone Medicines

It is logical to conclude that metformin might help manage hirsutism, through reductions in insulin-induced ovarian androgens and improvements in SHBG levels. Nevertheless, not many studies have been carried out to evaluate the specific effect of metformin. In general, based on studies that have been published, prolonged use of metformin is required to achieve modest improvements in unwanted hair growth. Also, metformin is not FDA-approved for the treatment of hirsutism. A 1995 study in the *Journal of Clinical Endocrinology and Metabolism* by Dr. J. C. Crave and colleagues in France found that metformin offered no significant improvement over nutritional changes, when comparing SHBG levels, androgen levels, and hirsutism in each group.

In a multicenter study published in 2001 in the same journal, Dr. Ricardo Azziz and colleagues found that troglitazone (Rezulin) offered a significant improvement in hirsutism scores after forty-four weeks, when compared to placebo. The study did not incorporate a comparative benefit of insulin-reducing life-management strategies. Furthermore, troglitazone has been withdrawn from the market, and it is not yet known if the other oral glitazone medications—

pioglitazone (Actos) and rosiglitazone (Avandia)—would offer a similar benefit. Some researchers have hypothesized that glitazone drugs might have a direct and positive effect on hair follicles and sebaceous glands by interfering with insulin and IGF-1 action. Future clinical research will be required to test this possibility.

HEAT AND LIGHT: TREATING THE HAIR THAT'S THERE

The medications and lifestyle strategies mentioned above can normalize free androgen levels in the bloodstream and block androgen action in the hair follicle, limiting the production of new, "active" follicles. Nevertheless, previously activated follicles will stubbornly defy those treatments and continue to produce hair. Definitive treatment of unwanted hair growth requires destruction of the cells within each individual active follicle. For many years, electrolysis was the only effective treatment. More recently, laser treatments have gained popularity as both competing and complementary options.

It's Easier to Call It Electrolysis

Electroepilation is the proper technical name for electrolysis, a procedure that was originally developed in the nineteenth century by Dr. Charles Michel. Dr. Michel's technique was first applied to ingrown eyelashes, with modifications later made for unwanted hair growth elsewhere on the face and body.

Electrolysis destroys the cells and vascular tissue that support the hair; once this occurs, each hair can be removed with sterile tweezers. There are currently three different methods utilized. The first is galvanic electrolysis, where a tiny needle is inserted into the hair follicle, and a direct current is applied. The second is called thermolysis, whereby the current in the needle produces destructive heat. Last, a blended technique combines galvanic and thermolytic procedures.

Electrolysis may be more effective for some women than others, depending on the location and quantity of unwanted hair they wish to have removed during the visit. Women typically describe the procedure as mildly uncomfortable during the time that current or heat is being applied to each hair follicle. However, oral analgesics ahead of time can help, and topical anesthetic creams containing lidocaine and prilocaine are commonly used during electrolysis. Shaving the areas you wish to have treated a few days before can improve effectiveness, since the electrologist can better find active follicles sprouting new hairs.

As with any cosmetic procedure, the skill of the operator is very important. Many communities have certified and licensed electrologists with good reputations who usually work independently, but may work under the auspices of a beauty salon, spa, or even in a physician's office. Since previously dormant hair follicles typically become activated to grow new hair, most women seek repeated treatments at time intervals under their discretion.

Societies such as the American Electrology Association (www.electrology.com) have recognized the fact that unwanted hair growth may be linked to hyperandrogenism, and have recommended that doctors and electrologists work together to improve the health and well-being of women. Many women seeking care from an electrologist would also benefit from medical evaluation for underlying androgen-related problems, including insulin overproduction, obesity, irregular menses, and infertility.

The Energy of Light

A vast array of scientific knowledge and physics forms the foundation of medical laser treatments, dating back to the work and theories of Albert Einstein. Over the past three decades, laser devices of all different shapes and sizes have permeated medical care. Dr. T. H. Maiman first described the ruby crystal laser in 1960, and that mode of energy now forms the basis of one FDA approved laser system (the EpiLaser) for unwanted hair growth. With the right energy source, laser light rapidly converts to localized heat when the light energy is absorbed by tissues, making its applicability to hair removal procedures very appealing.

Red colored light emitted by the EpiLaser is absorbed only by melanin pigments located in the hair and hair follicles. The laser light is usually pulsed for only a fraction of a second, which is long enough to treat about a half-inch area of hair follicles with laser thermal energy. The amount of time needed for treatment depends on the size of the area being treated, which can include virtually any part of the body, including the face. The EpiLaser instrument utilizes a cooling device that protects the surface of the skin and provides patient comfort during the procedure. Many women describe laser treatments as less uncomfortable than electrolysis. Topical anesthetic cream can also be used. Multiple treatments might be required, since the laser only eradicates hair in its active phase of growth. Surrounding skin should not generally be affected by energy focused on the hair and follicles. Laser hair removal may not be applicable to everyone. Ideally, the person seeking this type of treatment has dark hair and light skin. The laser light energy is better absorbed in dark hair, and light skin tends to keep the energy focused in the hair follicle. Individuals with dark or tan skin may acquire unsightly pigmentation changes if not properly counseled in advance. Reputable facilities will often recommend a "patch test" first to people with darker skin, to determine if the skin is at risk for permanent discoloration. Due to the possibility of temporary skin discoloration, many centers advise clients to schedule treatments more than one week prior to important social engagements. Electrolysis can serve as a complementary treatment to remove isolated hairs in between scheduled laser treatments.

Physicians who perform laser therapy are usually board-certified dermatologists or plastic surgeons. However, many licensed physicians, including family practice doctors, endocrinologists, and gynecologists, have learned the technique and now offer laser hair removal in their practices. Business arrangements between cosmetology centers and physicians are common and may provide the best of both worlds for women seeking a variety of cosmetic treatments at one time, or in the same location. "Buyer beware" is the best advice, since only capable and trained experts should carry out laser therapy. Market forces in any particular community may determine price and availability, and some centers offer financing.

Unusual But True—Hirsutism Unrelated to Syndrome O

Rapid development or worsening of hirsutism at any age can sometimes indicate a serious underlying condition, such as an androgen-producing tumor of the adrenal gland or ovary. Screening tests for such tumors include blood level measurements for testosterone, androstenedione, and DHEAS. Although quite rare, women are sometimes afraid to seek care for virilizing symptoms since they are fearful or embarrassed. With the onset of high androgen levels, menses and ovulation tend to cease. Modern imaging techniques of CT scan and MRI allow for rapid diagnosis of androgen-producing tumors, leading to accurate surgical treatment.

Excessively high cortisol levels (*hypercortisolism*) can be caused by adenomas in the pituitary gland (Cushing's disease), or by tumors in the adrenal gland and elsewhere in the body (Cushing's syndrome). These abnormalities cause the adrenal gland to overproduce cortisol in an uncontrolled fashion, and often adrenal androgens as well. Hypercortisolism typically leads to rapid weight gain, central obesity, hirsutism, and cessation of menses, thus mimicking certain features of polycystic ovaries and Syndrome O. Endocrinologists are usually on the lookout for hypercortisolism, and testing is warranted in certain clinical settings. Two screening tests are commonly carried out: 1) the twenty-four-hour urinary free cortisol test (the patient collects her urine for twenty-four hours and then turns it into a lab, where free cortisol is measured); and 2) the low dose dexamethasone suppression test (the patient is instructed to take a 1-milligram tablet of dexamethasone at 11 P.M., with a measurement of blood cortisol level taken at 8 A.M.) Additional hormone and imaging tests are usually required to locate the source of unregulated adrenal stimulation, with treatment instituted once the right diagnosis is made.

Inherited gene abnormalities in enzymes necessary for cortisol synthesis can contribute to high adrenal androgen production. Hirsutism and irregular menstrual cycles can result, but not usually obesity. Excess androgens from the adrenal gland can commonly interfere with normal ovarian function. Some cases of precocious puberty are linked to this problem. In adults, the most common adrenal enzyme blockade occurs in the 21-hydroxylase enzyme, which can cause a disorder called adult-onset congenital adrenal hyperplasia (CAH). A less common genetic enzyme block involves the 11-hydroxylase enzyme. Individuals affected by CAH produce inadequate quantities of cortisol, but excess amounts of androgens. Treatment usually requires that a cortisol-like medication, such as dexamethasone or prednisone, be taken indefinitely by affected individuals. There is some evidence that insulin overproduction may worsen the androgen impact of even mild CAH, since insulin stimulates androgen-producing enzymes in the adrenal gland.

Certain ethnic groups are at highest risk for CAH, including Ashkenazi Jews and certain individuals of Mediterranean descent. In New York City it has been estimated that at least 1 to 2 percent of women and men carry genes related to CAH. The best screening test for CAH involves checking 17-hydroxyprogesterone blood levels in the fasting state. If elevated, more detailed testing should be carried out, including DNA analysis for gene perturbations. Women who have adult-onset CAH are at risk for passing more severe forms of CAH to their children, particularly if their husbands or partners are genetic carriers. If pregnancy is desired, preconception genetic counseling is strongly recommended. During pregnancy, genetic testing is best carried out in the first trimester via chorionic villus sampling (which tests the placenta cells from a first-trimester pregnancy), although amniocentesis (which checks fetal cells in amniotic fluid in the second trimester) can also be used to make the diagnosis. Many states require neonatal testing. Fetuses inheriting severe CAH genes are at risk for virilization, along with ambiguous genitalia and life-threatening metabolic problems at birth. Fortunately, babies who are diagnosed with severe CAH by prenatal testing can usually be successfully treated *in utero* by administering higher doses of dexamethasone to the mother.

BEAUTIFUL INSIDE AND OUT: KEY MOTIVATIONAL POINTS

- All women have the freedom to pursue improvements in mind, body, and spirit. The desire for outward beauty and perfect appearance is never-ending for some people, leading to disappointment and emptiness. Women receive mixed signals about appearance from different aspects of society, including other women.
- Women with Syndrome O commonly have many different appearance issues to contend with, particularly related to the effects of insulin and androgen overproduction. Unwanted hair growth on the face and other parts of the body is a major appearance and beauty issue for many women.
- Although rare, women and their doctors should always be on the lookout for life-threatening virilization symptoms, which usually occur rapidly and create much more dramatic problems than hirsutism. Adrenal and ovarian tumors are usually the cause.
- Hirsutism is caused by elevations in free androgens, as well as the inherited sensitivity of hair follicles to many different hormones. Women with Syndrome O usually have elevated free androgens, as reflected by moderate increases in total ovarian and/or adrenal androgens and significant decreases in liver SHBG production. As such, androgen excess most often reflects a disordered metabolic state of insulin overproduction.
- Medications for prevention of hirsutism include many different brands of birth control pills, anti-androgens such as spirono-

lactone, the facial cream Vaniqa, GnRH agonists, and possibly insulin-sensitizing drugs. Lifestyle management, as described by the SOS Strategies, can only help with prevention efforts.

- Electrolysis has been the mainstay for permanent hair removal, although laser hair removal is rapidly gaining popularity. Certain skin colors and hair characteristics may make laser treatments unwise for some women. Costs can be prohibitive for many people. Women who seek care for hair removal should also consider medical evaluation for androgen excess and insulin overproduction.

- Less common causes of hirsutism include virilizing tumors of the adrenal gland and ovary, hypercortisolism caused by Cushing's disease or syndrome, and adult-onset congenital adrenal hyperplasia. These diseases are treatable and may have implications prior to and during pregnancy.

ELEVEN

MAMAS AND PAPAS, CYSTERS AND BROTHERS: MEAN GENES FOR MODERN TIMES

THOSE DARN ABNORMAL GENES: THE CONTROVERSY CONTINUES

Many in the medical community believe that women with Syndrome O have defective genes. Billions of dollars from the federal government and the pharmaceutical industry have been invested in the defective gene concept for common metabolic-related disorders, such as type 2 diabetes, obesity, heart disease, hypertension, and even polycystic ovaries. While there is no doubt that new scientific knowledge is constantly needed to understand how our genes work, could research dollars be better spent improving our crippled metabolic environment?

The structure of DNA was discovered over fifty years ago by Nobel laureates Drs. James Watson, Francis Crick, and Maurice Wilkins (Dr. Rosalind Franklin was equally credited, but died of ovarian cancer before the Nobel prize was awarded). Soon after, scientists learned that DNA within genes is very dependably replicated from one cell generation to the next. Genetic "drift" requires the passing of thousands of generations, meaning that alterations in DNA and genes occur very gradually. Small or large changes in DNA and genes—called *mutations*—can either help or hurt subsequent generations and the survivability of a species.

The diversity of mankind reflects a subtle genetic drift that spanned thousands of years, leading to ethnic differences in outward appearance and the inner functioning of tissues and organs. Although every human being has a unique DNA "fingerprint" based on the spacing of genes throughout the chromosomes, genes that control metabolism and reproduction are actually quite similar from one person to the next. It is safe to assume that modern mankind's genes have hardly changed from those of our Paleolithic and Neolithic ancestors. Furthermore, no matter where on the planet your ancestors may have come from, they likely had outstanding genes for instructing the body how to digest food, metabolize calories, and reproduce. You are here now because they survived and reproduced way back when.

Hybrid vigor—gaining genetic strength from one's biological mother and father—is a basic tenet of reproduction. The concept dates back to the 1860s, when an Austrian monk named Gregor Mendel carried out breeding experiments with pea plants. In humans, prospective parents often share cultural or ethnic backgrounds. However, all humans are sufficiently unique to provide hybrid vigor to each successive generation, following patterns of Mendelian genetics. Some gene mutations have been present in families for many generations, leading to true genetic diseases, such as cystic fibrosis, sickle cell anemia, and Tay Sachs disease. Fortunately, most mutations causing disease are carried as *recessive* traits and appear relatively infrequently as full-blown disease. Cystic fibrosis is one of the most common recessive gene abnormalities known, with one normal and one abnormal gene appearing in about 4 percent of Caucasians. Even with that relatively high carrier frequency, the actual chances of a child being born with cystic fibrosis is only about one in 2,500, or 0.04 percent.

Many dominant traits are lethal, and commonly adulthood is not reached to pass a dominant trait on to the next generation. Huntingdon's disease is one example. Sex-linked genetic diseases, such as hemophilia, are carried on the X chromosome and are most likely to affect males, who only have one X chromosome. Recessive, dominant, and sex-linked diseases are usually due to specific and identifiable gene mutations or rearrangements—also called *polymorphisms*—in affected individuals. Modern science has made tremendous strides in identifying gene mutations and polymorphisms that *directly* cause or predict numerous life-threatening and life-debilitating diseases.

One popular field of exploration among medical scientists has been to measure inherited *propensity* for disease, based on patterns of genes within families. Some abnormal gene patterns or mutations predict the onset of serious diseases with a high degree of certainty, such as cancer and early age heart disease. A strong family history is usually present as well. Other gene patterns are less predictive, such as those that contribute to diabetes and obesity. The use of modern molecular biology to predict future disease has pluses and minuses in the eyes of medical ethicists and the public.

While prevention of disease is an important mission of medical research, we are all mortals and will likely succumb to some disease sooner or later. Knowing one's genetic destiny for a particular disease could help with prevention, but there is significant concern about potential discrimination and abuse. A belief that one's health destiny is predetermined may also lead to a diminution of personal responsibility, i.e. "I just have to pray that those scientists find my abnormal genes."

The Paradox of Modern Living

Could our perfectly normal genes be malfunctioning in a world of overnourishment and underactivity? Do unnatural funny fats and sugary processed foods add fuel to the fire? Do we have free will, or is our fate completely predetermined by genetics and environment? At what point can environment, societal expectations, and personal decisions from day to day overwhelm our genetic destiny?

In the United States, we live in a society that paradoxically desires a high quality of life, yet is willing to accept a risk for unprecedented amounts of disease. Although life expectancy continues to rise in the United States, disorders associated with metabolic dysfunction are increasingly chipping away at our health, quality of life, and fertility. The evidence for this assertion is based on an eye-opening review of what experts knew less than a century ago about problems like diabetes and polycystic ovaries.

Diabetes and Our Genetic "Flaws"

Endocrinologists of the 1930s had very sophisticated knowledge about diabetes. In 1936, Dr. William Wolf expressed concern that the incidence and death rate of diabetes in the United States had risen more rapidly than any other disease. "It is fair to assume that there are constantly from 270,000 to 300,000 diabetic patients in the United States," it was stated in his book *Endocrinology in Modern Practice*. The American Diabetes Association now estimates that there are at least *16 million people* in the United States with type 2 diabetes. Although the population of the United States has increased about 2.3-fold since the 1930s, the number of diabetics has increased 50- to 60-fold.

In the 1930s, the greatest increase in prevalence of diabetes was attributed to women, with a 117 percent increase since 1910. Overall, about 1 adult in 350 to 500 had diabetes in 1936. Now, *1 person in 15* has diabetes, including millions of children, adolescents, and young adults.

Regarding women and the modern risk of diabetes, recall the results from the study, in which one in twenty-six nurses developed diabetes during a sixteen-year time period in the 1980s and '90s. Many more of those 85,000 women had ongoing risk factors, and the final tally of diabetes among that group of women is not yet known.

Dr. Wolf noted that "diabetes affects the higher rather than the lower social strata" and that it is seen "least frequently in those whose occupations involve hard manual labor." The implication is that physical work and exertion protected people from developing diabetes, even in 1936. When easier availability of food and drink became matched up with a less active lifestyle, some good metabolic genes began to malfunction. Perhaps the growing usage and convenience of the automobile was also contributory.

The important lesson to be learned is that compared to now, diabetes was relatively uncommon. And before the 1930s, it was even rarer. Many scientists now are looking for abnormal genes that cause diabetes. Is that logical? Obviously, many things in our environment have changed in the past one hundred years, including our food quality and quantity, our propensity for underactivity, and the epidemic of obesity. In my opinion, it really doesn't make sense to spend one more dime looking for abnormal genes.

What About the Genes That Cause Syndrome O and Polcystic Ovaries?

The original Stein-Leventhal syndrome was based on case reports involving only *seven women,* archived over a number of years while the two doctors were practicing gynecology in Chicago. Even though they removed large portions of ovaries from these women, no diseased tissue was ever found. As they reported, "The pathologist is unable to conclude from a study of the sections taken from the ovaries in our patients that amenorrhea [lack of periods] was a symptom. He can demonstrate no anatomic structure or characteristic change in the ovary which enables him to describe the clinical picture. The only consistent pathologic finding is the presence of follicle cysts lined by theca cells."

Dr. Wolf considered the possibility in 1936 that diabetes in women had some link with sterility and lack of menstrual cycles. He thought that insulin might be involved. Nevertheless, the insulin-ovary connection hardly garnered any attention from gynecologists, since a syndrome of polycystic ovaries barely existed in the 1930s. Women who had diabetes in 1936 were usually overweight, yet only mildly so by today's standards.

As the twenty-first century unfolds, Syndrome O is now a major contributing factor to infertility and other gynecologic problems. The exact number of women suffering with Syndrome O is not known, but estimates exceed five million in the United States. Clearly, neither diabetes nor Syndrome O are hidden epidemics. Have the genes of our parents, or parents' parents become abnormal in just a few generations? From our sophisticated knowledge about genes and DNA, we know that just isn't possible.

Perhaps scientists would be better off studying how our genes function in the New Age of overnourishment and underactivity. Based on the historical facts, philosophical arguments, and common sense, only you can decide what you wish to believe about your genes.

ARE YOU MY MOTHER?

Few can forget P. D. Eastman's poignant classic childhood tale, which described the educational wanderings of an inquisitive newly hatched bird while Mother looked for food. Many Syndrome O women have embarked on similar inquiring journeys, eager to understand why their metabolism and fertility differ so greatly from that of their mothers and grandmothers. The answers lie in understanding how normal genes are inherited and how these genes might function in less-than-optimal settings.

Insulin Versus Ovaries

From a geneticist's viewpoint, Syndrome O could be viewed as a battleground of many genes inherited from both mother and father. Two significant groups of genes are relevant: Great Gene Set #1: those promoting thrifty, efficient metabolism; and Great Gene Set #2: those responsible for sensitive, fertile ovaries. All people who inherit Great Gene Set #1 will be at risk for insulin overproduction *if* they are overnourished. The challenge of avoiding overnourishment is magnified dramatically if Great Gene Set #1 is inherited from both parents! Chronic overnourishment will quickly overwhelm thrifty metabolic genes, leading to excessive lipogenesis, weight gain, obesity, and insulin resistance. If insulin overproduction becomes chronic, other diseases of the metabolic syndrome will result for both women and men.

Women who inherit Great Gene Sets #1 and #2 from one or both parents are genetically programmed to *potentially* develop insulin overproduction, ovarian confusion, and ovulation disruption—i.e., Syndrome O. The severity of overnourishment and the extent of insulin overproduction will directly affect the action of sensitive, fertile ovaries. Throughout history, genetically enhanced women inherited *both* Great Gene Sets #1 and #2, allowing them to survive scarce food sources and to reproduce efficiently when insulin levels were low.

Many overnourished and overweight women have inherited Great Gene Set #1, yet do not typically manifest all of the clinical symptoms of Syndrome O and polycystic ovaries. Without Great Gene Set #2,

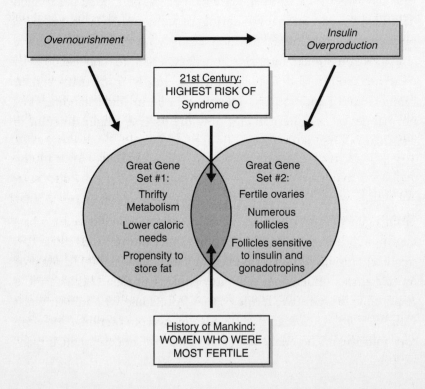

their ovaries may not be particularly sensitive to excess insulin. Their ovaries may or may not overproduce androgens, but they often have excess free androgens. They often ovulate and conceive without fertility treatments. Nevertheless, overnourished and obese women who conceive on their own are at risk for other significant reproductive problems, including miscarriage and high-risk pregnancies. They should be considered in the spectrum of Syndrome O because they also have significant risks for metabolic disorders and may eventually develop ovarian confusion and ovulation disruption.

Other women can inherit just Great Gene Set #2, leading to the so-called thin polycystic ovary disorder. Although thinner women with polycystic ovaries may not have overt weight or metabolic problems, their bodies are still overproducing insulin relative to the amount required by their ovaries. The proof for this is that ovulation and pregnancy can occur in these women when they utilize insulin-lowering strategies. Depending on the sensitivity of their uterus, blood vessels, and clotting systems to excess insulin, they may also suffer from other reproductive problems. Later in life they may still develop metabolic disorders and may become overweight and insulin resistant.

From a practical viewpoint, Syndrome O women can have mothers who were either thin or not-so-thin. A thin mother probably had relatively sensitive ovaries, since she was able to ovulate and reproduce successfully in a setting of lower insulin levels. A not-so-thin mother may have reproduced successfully because she had less sensitive ovaries, even if her insulin levels were high. Unless your mother had overt Syndrome O and/or polycystic ovaries, it is hard to know for sure how sensitive her ovaries actually were. However, it is a fact that many fewer women had Syndrome O before 1980.

Most Syndrome O women I've met report that their mothers were fertile, whether thin or not-so-thin. Furthermore, Syndrome O women usually have siblings, permitting some interesting scientific observations to be made concerning the impact of insulin overproduction within families. One thing is certain—your mother must have been reasonably fertile to sprout the egg that brought you into the world.

Many Syndrome O women—perhaps as many as 50 percent or more—appear to inherit features of gene set #1 primarily from their fathers. A detailed family history often demonstrates some significant aspects of Syndrome X on the father's side of the family, including aunts, uncles, and grandparents. As expected, a paternal family history of obesity, diabetes, heart disease, hypertension, dyslipidemias, and even premature baldness is commonly identified when taking a detailed family history from Syndrome O women. To what extent sensitive and fertile ovaries—gene set #2—can be inherited from the father's side of the family is hard to know. However, Syndrome O women usually report that their paternal grandmothers were fertile; it's also rare that their fathers are without siblings.

CYSTERS AND THEIR BROTHERS

In the early 1980s, medical scientists started revisiting the concept that the ovaries could be affected by insulin overproduction. Although gynecologists Drs. Stein and Leventhal didn't make this connection, it was originally proposed in the 1930s by some shrewd endocrinologists. With the burst of technology in modern molecular biology starting in the 1980s, scientists began to explore relationships between genes and common diseases, particularly diabetes and heart disease.

Dr. Andrea Dunaif is considered a pioneer in the search for genes and genetic factors potentially associated with polycystic ovaries. One landmark study published in 1995 in the *Journal of Clinical Investigation* opened the door to the possibility that Syndrome O women may have a unique profile of insulin action within their connective tissue and skeletal muscle. When insulin acted upon their tissues, biochemical differences were observed in the function of the insulin receptor. Dr. Dunaif has proposed that this same biochemical problem could also occur in the ovaries, leading to androgen overproduction. It is still not known if this finding represents a true congenital abnormality in genes regulating insulin action, or a gradual malfunctioning of otherwise normal genes. Thus far, no specific gene mutations have been identified, and Dr. Dunaif has suggested that insulin resistance itself might unmask this problem.

The hunt for the purported "PCOS gene" (or genes) continues. In 2001, Dr. Stefania Tucci and colleagues at Mt. Sinai School of Medicine in New York identified a region of DNA near the insulin receptor gene that was found more commonly in women with poly-cystic ovaries. Of ten different DNA markers studied in close prox-imity to the insulin receptor gene, only one—D19S884—appeared relevant to their search. The results were published in the *Journal of Clinical Endocrinology and Metabolism*. Previous work in 1999 by Dr. Margrit Urbanek and colleagues at the University of Pennsylvania had also raised the possibility of a linkage to this same "hot spot," marker D19S884, but their results were not statistically significant.

The higher prevalence of insulin overproduction, androgen ex-cess, and polycystic ovaries within many families is now well known. However, the work of Dr. Richard Legro and colleagues at Penn State Hershey Medical School, the University of Pennsylvania, and Harvard University were instrumental in establishing this fact. In one study, the sisters of eighty women with confirmed polycystic ovaries were closely evaluated. Approximately one half of the sisters had no evidence of polycystic ovaries or elevated androgen levels. However, 22 percent of the sisters had abnormal menstrual cycles with elevated androgens (the NIH definition of PCOS), while 24 percent had reg-ular menses with elevated androgens. Interestingly, the PCOS women and their affected sisters had a markedly elevated average BMI of 33 to 34. The sisters with elevated androgens and regular menses had an average BMI of 29; unaffected sisters had an average BMI of 26. Two sets of genes appear to have been inherited independently in this group of women: one set regulating metabolism and weight, and an-other set controlling ovarian sensitivity to insulin.

Another landmark study by Dr. A. Govind and colleagues at the Keele University in the United Kingdom evaluated the inheritance pattern of polycystic ovaries within families and the extent to which both female *and* male family members were affected. Their findings, published in 1999 in the *Journal of Clinical Endocrinology and Metabolism,* were startling. In twenty-nine families where women had polycystic ovaries on ultrasound and/or elevated blood androgen levels, thirty-five of fifty-three sisters (61 percent) were also affected. In addition, six of twenty-eight fathers (21 percent) and four of eighteen brothers (22 percent) were found to have severe premature balding before the age of thirty. Balding is closely related to insulin overproduction and excess free androgens, leading to excess DHT in the hair follicles of the scalp. Thus, it appears that "PCOS genes" could be affecting a substantial number of men also.

It has been suggested that if men developed polycystic testicles as part of male Syndrome X, medical scientists might pay closer attention. Of interest, it is suspected that sperm count and sperm quality in men with diabetes, obesity, and severe insulin resistance may be impaired, although this possibility requires further investigation.

Scientists committed to researching the genetics of Syndrome O realize that they might not find any abnormal genes. However, they may find important DNA regions that are associated with various dysfunctional aspects of insulin overproduction and ovarian sensitivity. Whether this provides useful information for the prevention of disease remains to be determined. An extensive and thorough up-to-date review regarding the molecular biology of polycystic ovaries was co-authored in 2002 by Dr. Legro at Penn State Hershey and Dr. Jerome Strauss at the University of Pennsylvania. In their article, published in *Fertility and Sterility,* they note that existing research suggests strongly that polycystic ovaries tend to cluster in families, and that ovarian cells and fat tissue from such women may function differently when compared to women without polycystic ovaries. They believe there may be genes linked to susceptibility of Syndrome O, but that the function of these genes are possibly modified by environmental factors. Furthermore, they state: "The fact that genetic studies have not yet pinpointed a polycystic ovary syndrome locus or mutation should not be disheartening news. The search is still in its infancy, and studies of adequate power and design to identify genes are under way."

Rather than blame bad or diseased genes, I believe it is more credible to assume that millions of women with Syndrome O—from every corner of the world and from every ethnic group—have wonderful "designer" genes. Such genes have promoted thrifty metabolism and efficient reproduction throughout the world and through the ages for thousands of years. Learning how normal genes malfunction in an environment of overnourishment and insulin overproduction might be a more rewarding journey for scientists now and in the future.

PRECOCIOUS, BUT NOT SO CUTE— KEEPING AN "I" ON THE KIDS

Many Syndrome O women remember a troubling problem of their childhood—early puberty. More recently, increasing numbers of young girls are experiencing *precocious*—or very early—puberty, with the onset of pubic and axillary hair, breast development, and even menstrual cycles prior to the age of eight. Although not considered abnormal by many doctors, early puberty at age nine or ten may also be met with significant concern, particularly if menstrual patterns are abnormal. Some experts suspect that the insulin family of hormones is the culprit in this trend toward early puberty, leading to inappropriately early "wake-up" signals in the brain-pituitary-ovary glandular internet.

An epidemic of childhood obesity is clearly correlated with insulin overproduction and an alarming increase in the incidence of diabetes in young people. In 1996, Dr. O. Pinhas-Hamiel and colleagues at the Cincinnati Children's Hospital reported in the *Journal of Pediatrics* that the incidence of adolescent non-insulin-dependent diabetes *increased tenfold* in Cincinnati over a twelve-year period from 1982 to 1994. Among those adolescents diagnosed, the average body mass index was 38, in the markedly obese range. Of particular note, female patients were typically diagnosed one year earlier in age than males, and 63 percent of the new adolescent diabetes cases were female.

Most of the young diabetics evaluated in this study had a parent or sibling previously diagnosed with diabetes, suggesting a strong inheritance pattern. Thrifty genes, when throttled by overnourishment and inactivity, do not appear to have any ethnic, racial, or age boundaries.

In 2003, the American Heart Association released a scientific statement, written as an article by Drs. Julia Steinberger and Stephen Daniels in the journal *Circulation,* which discussed the interrelationships between obesity, insulin resistance, diabetes, and cardiovascular risk in children. Their position was reviewed and endorsed by the American Diabetes Association. They found that the "increase in frequency of type 2 diabetes seems to parallel the increase in prevalence and severity of obesity in children and adolescents."

Numerous physicians and researchers in pediatric specialties are taking note of the links between adolescent insulin overproduction in girls, premature or early puberty, and the subsequent development of polycystic ovaries. An expression of concern is clearly growing in the medical literature, particularly in view of the frightening increase in adolescent diabetes since the 1980s.

Genetic tendencies for early onset Syndrome O are clearly related to inheritance patterns of the thrifty metabolism gene set #1 and sensitive fertile ovary gene set #2. One of the biggest concerns related to adolescent Syndrome O is the fact that young women's ovaries are particularly susceptible to insulin and LH. An adolescent's ovaries contain many more dormant follicles than a woman in her twenties or thirties. A theoretical concern is that the infertility aspects of Syndrome O may be even harder to overcome in the future as insulin overproduction worsens in adolescent girls. Prevention strategies are vital but pose more of a challenge.

Women who are seeking fertility care and a healthy pregnancy are likely to be very motivated to institute effective insulin-reducing strategies. Can adolescents be just as motivated? Dr M. E. Trent and colleagues at Johns Hopkins University School of Medicine addressed quality-of-life attitudes among ninety-seven adolescent girls with polycystic ovaries. In one publication in 2002, in the *Archives of*

Pediatrics and Adolescent Medicine, it was noted that the ninety-seven girls scored lower than control subjects in areas of general health perceptions, physical functioning, general behavior, and limitations in family activities. The authors suggest that there is a strong need to develop interventions for reducing the distress these girls may face as adolescents and young adults. In a second publication in 2003 by the same authors, in the *Journal of Pediatric and Adolescent Gynecology,* they reported that the ninety-seven girls expressed particular concern about their future fertility. They were 3.4 times more likely to be worried about getting pregnant in the future (as adults!) when compared to a control group of adolescent girls.

Where can teens with Syndrome O turn for help? The SOS Strategies described earlier can provide a useful framework for getting started. With parental guidance, adolescents can hopefully pursue the initial steps of education, motivation, and stimulation in an environment that is supportive and nonjudgmental. A knowledgeable and compassionate adolescent gynecologist, pediatrician, or endocrinologist should closely evaluate adolescents with symptoms of Syndrome O. Both metabolic and reproductive aspects should be assessed, and a treatment plan should take into account ongoing issues of insulin overproduction and irregular menstrual cycles. Future work will need to determine the applicability of the SOS Strategies for adolescents. Nevertheless, it seems likely that young women could benefit greatly from an organized and optimized approach to time management, nutrition, exercise, stress reduction, and the pursuit of happiness.

MAKING YOUR GENES WORK FOR YOU: KEY MOTIVATIONAL POINTS

- Our metabolic and reproductive genes functioned quite well through generations of mankind, spanning hundreds of thousands of years. Laws of genetics dictate that our genes haven't changed very much over the years. Hybrid vigor should only make them stronger.

- Scientists are now analyzing genes to determine human propensity for developing certain diseases. Often the same level of predictability can be determined through detailed family history. Knowing one's fate based on genetic analysis may or may not be useful for preventing disease.

- The incidence of diabetes in the United States has risen sharply over the past one hundred years, suggesting that the major culprit is environmental, not genetic. Current epidemics of obesity, overnourishment, and underactivity hardly existed in the earlier part of the twentieth century. Some shrewd endocrinologists in the 1930s were alerted to the mounting problem of diabetes and obesity, which has only worsened dramatically since that time.

- From a genetic perspective, most women with Syndrome O probably inherited two great sets of genes: 1) those that promote a thrifty, low-calorie metabolic existence; and 2) those that provide the ovaries with numerous insulin and gonadotropin-sensitive follicles. Throughout the history of mankind, women with both gene sets were the most metabolically fit and probably the most fertile.

- Abnormal genes or gene mutations related to polycystic ovaries have not been found. However, normal metabolic and reproductive genes may be malfunctioning in an environment of overnourishment and insulin overproduction. Clusters of families have "PCOS genes," which contribute to obesity and androgen excess in women *and* men. Men manifest androgen excess through premature balding and possibly with decreases in sperm count and quality.

- The epidemic of overnourishment is spreading to children and adolescents at an alarming rate. The metabolic consequences are severe obesity at an early age and early onset of glucose intolerance, insulin overproduction, and diabetes. The ovaries and reproductive system of adolescent girls are particularly sensitive to the effects of insulin overproduction.

- Early or precocious puberty, along with irregular menses, can be predictive for the later development of Syndrome O. They could be markers for insulin overproduction during childhood. Evaluation by adolescent medical professionals in conjunction with strategic lifestyle interventions is highly recommended.
- Never let your genes get in your way. Always give yourself a fighting chance. You'll be a winner each and every day.

TWELVE

LESA'S STORY: EMPOWERMENT BY HEALING SYNDROME O

A Child Is Born

You wouldn't suspect anything unusual about Lesa, or her fertility challenges, if you caught a glimpse of her shuttling three kids in a minivan on the mountain roads near Asheville, North Carolina. Like many other women, Lesa performs a sophisticated juggling act between work, school, church, chores, home life, and volunteer time as a nonprofit corporate CEO. Despite a hectic day-to-day pace, Lesa maintains classic Southern poise, charm, and a wry sense of humor. Her friends say, "Bless her heart, she's never been happier." Lesa is a Syndrome O survivor.

"A few years ago I didn't think I came from a particularly 'good egg,'" notes Lesa. "My mother is thin and in her childbearing years was very fertile. Her mother had ten children! For years, I wondered why I was so different from my mother and grandmother." Lesa also assumed that some horrible genetic twist of fate was causing her ovaries to become diseased and her fertility to be impaired. Since doctors didn't seem to have any specific answers or advice, she suffered in silence.

The birth of her first baby symbolized a culmination of incredible efforts by one woman who successfully met the challenges of Syndrome O. Most significantly, the partnership Lesa established with her fertility specialist sparked the marvel of baby Hannah's conception, and possibly the creation of a new health movement. Each of the miracle Childers kids—Elizabeth, Hannah, and Daniel—have unique lessons to teach women, as well as their loving partners, who are grappling with Syndrome O and infertility.

Origins of Lesa's Syndrome O

Lesa is not shy about describing the symptoms of Syndrome O that she developed as a teenager—absent menstrual periods, dramatic weight gain, undesired hair growth on her face and body, and rapidly worsening body image and self-esteem. When looking back at her adolescent years, Lesa notes:

> I really ate poorly, and I certainly didn't get any exercise. Even now I have a hard time thinking about how I looked and felt.
>
> I began having irregular periods at the age of eleven, and my mother just assumed that was normal. My mother, who is thinner, didn't start having periods until she was sixteen, and they were regular. During my yearly physicals, I would tell the pediatrician that my periods were abnormal—often skipping months, then bleeding heavily for several days. We were always told that this was normal for girls my age, and that it would correct itself with time. This continued until I was eighteen.
>
> Finally, I called our family physician after skipping my period for a whole year and demanded that something had to be done. I generally felt horrible and knew that something wasn't right. By this time, I weighed over 180 pounds and had developed hair growth on my face. The doctor put me on birth control pills to regulate my periods, but the

very first month I was on the pills I had a horrible bleeding experience. I hemorrhaged for two straight weeks; it was so bad that I couldn't attend school for a week. The doctor who prescribed the pills instructed me to take extra pills each day, but she offered no explanation for the heavy bleeding. Gradually, my periods became more regular, and I assumed that with the birth control pill, my problems were solved. I now know the pill was just a Band-Aid.

You wouldn't have recognized me then. I was sluggish and poorly focused. I believe I was bright and opinionated, but just didn't have the same outlook on life that I do now. I was miserable in my own skin. My dad said to me once, "You had better use your brain because who is going to hire you based on your looks?" I didn't know what to do with my intelligence. It's like the real me was hidden beneath the fat. My dad's rejection of my physical self was very hard on me. I've never liked disappointing my father. When I couldn't be the slim beauty queen he expected me to be, I just gave up trying. I wore baggy clothes, avoided makeup, and let my hair grow wild and unstyled. My parents were very embarrassed by me. Looking back, I'm convinced I became clinically depressed. My body was out of control and I really had no idea how to help myself.

When I finally started to get answers in my late twenties, I began my lifestyle change. With weight loss came enhanced pride in myself, and the transformation to the "real me" gradually began. I peeled off layer after layer of my protective mask. It became safe for me to feel attractive and OK about my body, even though it was far from perfect. I reversed the vicious cycle of negativity; that still feels great!

Adding to Lesa's initial confusion about her problems was the fact that her mother and grandmothers were thin in their younger years, and quite fertile. However, that was in an era when men and women shared plenty of hard, physically demanding work. While Lesa was growing up, food was more plentiful, but caloric burn and activity were not. Foods were commonly prepared in faster, processed "modern" ways (out of boxes, as frozen dinners, and with lots of partially hydrogenated funny fats). For years, Lesa wondered how she could have inherited such "bad genes" from her healthier and more fertile parents and grandparents.

Desperately Seeking Answers

With an inquiring and energetic mind, Lesa started looking for some legitimate answers to her menstrual problems when she got married over fifteen years ago. Initially there weren't many to find. One doctor told Lesa she might have an adrenal gland problem, prompting her to spend hours at the library reading about rare and horrible adrenal gland conditions. Fortunately, Lesa did not have any of these unusual or life-threatening diseases, but in her research she stumbled upon information related to polycystic ovary syndrome. Older information in the library indicated that this was also a relatively rare problem, causing missed periods, excess androgens, enlarged ovaries, and infertility. For Lesa, having an ovarian disease didn't seem any more palatable. Furthermore, there was little information to explain how polycystic ovaries arise in some women but not others, and virtually no information linking metabolism and lifestyle to the disorder.

Lesa notes: "I grew up in a very isolated environment. Mountain people who have been here for generations tend to distrust new information and are perfectly happy to remain blissfully ignorant of the outside world. However, the fact that I grew more physically unattractive in my teen years definitely affected my aspirations. While I was a part of the 'intellectual gang' at school, (participating in things like the newspaper and yearbook staff), I was not a popular girl. I married Lyle when I was eighteen, and he was obviously very tolerant of my quirkiness. After we married, it took us about two years to decide that we wanted children. I was working on a college degree part time, but I wanted it all . . . and fast."

From her research, Lesa initially concluded that her ovarian "disease" was going to completely thwart her chances of ever having a baby. Fertility treatments seemed to be a daunting and expensive prospect, fraught with risks of multiple pregnancy at one extreme, and downright failure as the sad alternative. Being poked and prodded by a fertility doctor on a frequent basis was also very unappealing, particularly when she already had great insecurity about her body image and weight. With all of these issues carefully considered, Lesa and her husband Lyle adopted their first child, Elizabeth.

"At that time, my doctors weren't giving me encouraging information about my fertility options," states Lesa. "And I was sick and tired of being made to feel like a freak. There is still a lot of misinformation and incomplete facts being given to women about polycystic ovaries and fertility. It is easy to assume now that women and their doctors understand these problems, since information is more readily available. But most women with Syndrome O aren't seeing reproductive endocrinologists and fertility experts. Most are seeking help from their primary care physicians and/or ob/gyns. Women often are not diagnosed thoroughly, and too often they are not informed of the potential seriousness of the metabolic disorder related to their reproductive health. I think many women still aren't aware that overnourishment, skipped menstrual periods, and unwanted hair could be very related problems. Often the symptoms are masked by birth control pills. I believe the key is getting information about polycystic ovaries and Syndrome O into the mainstream for millions of women who haven't yet learned about the connections."

The Diabetes Jolt

To complicate matters, Lesa developed type 2 diabetes at age twenty-eight. One of Lesa's friends, a nurse, noticed her flaming red cheeks, mood swings, and loss of energy. At that time Lesa weighed seventy-five pounds over her ideal body weight, with a body mass index (BMI) of 32, squarely in the obese range. A single fingerstick blood test performed by her friend revealed Lesa's blood sugar level to be 244 just two hours after eating, when normal levels should be under 140. Additional testing would confirm the diagnosis. Lesa now as-

sumed she had acquired another awful disease, which sent her back to
the library, to more doctors, and also to the Internet.

Shaken by the diabetes diagnosis, Lesa quickly learned that her
whole body was in a horrible state of insulin overdrive, with her pancreas being overstressed. Insulin overproduction had likely been going
on in her body for years, but as her muscles became even more resistant to insulin, extra glucose circulated in her bloodstream after meals
and even when fasting. Lesa was chronically tired, always moody, and
generally felt lousy for months. Her liver also went into revolt as her
lipogenic enzymes were producing fats and cholesterol at a furious
pace. Lesa's liver production of lipids was so high that some of the fat
could not escape to the bloodstream, a problem termed fatty liver.

Even with the two diagnoses of diabetes and polycystic ovaries,
Lesa's comprehension of the link wasn't obvious at first to either herself or her doctors. However, the word "diabetes" jolted Lesa, and she
points to the time her diabetes was diagnosed as a significant turning
point in her life. She became determined to treat her diabetes through
major changes in nutrition and exercise.

States Lesa: "I always thought of type 2 diabetes as an 'old person's
disease,' and to be afflicted with it at age twenty-eight was an eye
opener. Plus, with soaring lipid levels in my blood, I felt I was only a
few years away from a major blockage of coronary arteries that had
recently affected my forty-nine-year-old dad. Lifestyle change was
the only thing that made sense to me to avoid the double-whammy
dangers of diabetes and heart disease. My primary care doctor confirmed the fear I was expressing about my future health."

Although Dr. Sam Thatcher has previously characterized polycystic ovaries as a "hidden epidemic" in the title of his book, there is
nothing hidden about diabetes. In 1998, when Lesa's diabetes was first
uncovered, about 15 million other Americans had the same problem.
Diabetes continues to drain our nation's health-care dollars and psy-
che, and the incidence continues to soar. In 2003, the American Diabetes Association estimated that 17 million people in the United
States had diabetes. More concerning, it is believed that one-third of
those individuals had not been evaluated, diagnosed, or treated.

Like many people diagnosed with diabetes, Lesa instituted some dramatic strategic changes in her life. "For the first time ever, I took nutritional advice and the encouragement to exercise seriously. I had been offered and read about diet plans before, but suddenly I was motivated to learn on my own how to eat in a healthy way. I also learned that exercise was the key to controlling my blood sugars and insulin resistance. I developed my own plan for overcoming diabetes by reading as much as I could about the condition, talking to diabetes educators, learning from other diabetics, and eventually meeting with a reproductive endocrinologist. I experimented with different combinations of foods to determine how they affected my blood sugars. I tested my blood sugars compulsively. By keeping my blood sugars under control, I found that I felt much better and that my weight began to fall off. I made educated guesses about what would work for me and I kept on trying. I saw each day as an opportunity to reverse the damage that overnourishment had previously done to my body."

Many of Lesa's experiences mirror what other women have found through their own trials and tribulations. The Syndrome O Survival (SOS) Strategies were developed, and *Healing Syndrome O* was written, for millions of other women who don't know how to get started overcoming the challenges they face. Lesa now works closely with many women as she heads a 501(c)3 national nonprofit organization—PCOStrategies—with the mission of educating and motivating women to proactively heal Syndrome O.

In addition to the impact that diabetes had on her resolve to change key aspects of her life, Lesa was strongly motivated to become pregnant. Countless other women in the United States and around the world share this strong desire for a healthy pregnancy and child. Fortunately, 80 to 90 percent of women with Syndrome O will not be found to have diabetes in their twenties. However, if Syndrome O is ignored, most are at risk for developing it during pregnancy or later in life. As Lesa started her search for an experienced and caring fertility specialist, she would soon learn how closely her diabetes, Syndrome O, and infertility were linked.

THE INFERTILITY "BUNNY HOP"

Like many other women, Lesa's quest to have a baby started as a gnawing desire. Knowing that her reproductive system wasn't functioning properly, Lesa found a fertility specialist in Asheville, North Carolina, who seemed quite knowledgeable about her condition. That physician was Dr. Steve Sawin, a friend and colleague with whom I had worked at the University of Pennsylvania in the mid-1990s. "When I first met with Dr. Sawin," states Lesa, "he explained the link between my metabolic challenges and infertility. Another light then went off inside of my head. Finally, I had an answer to the question I had been asking myself and other doctors for years—'Why is my whole body, including my reproductive system, out of control?' I became even more motivated to continue my lifestyle program. There was really a chance for me to become pregnant if I could get my health and metabolism under control."

Armed with new knowledge and hope, and an excellent fertility practice rallying for her success, Lesa hopped on the roller coaster of fertility treatments for many months. Despite her initial enthusiasm she came very close to giving up, since numerous trials of ovulation induction were not resulting in success. Years of insulin overproduction had caused some serious changes in Lesa's ovaries. "My husband and I had a fertility budget of sorts, both with our finances and emotions," notes Lesa. "We were very reluctant to consider IVF if other treatments proved unsuccessful."

Although Dr. Sawin knew that there were thousands of healthy eggs housed in Lesa's two ovaries, every trick he had learned to induce ovulation with clomiphene and/or gonadotropins was being stymied. "I'm a walking textbook of how nasty insulin can be to your ovaries and your fertility, not to mention the rest of your body," states Lesa. Part of Lesa's eventual success may be related to the laparoscopic ovarian drilling procedure Dr. Sawin performed in 1998. As described in chapter 5, the rationale of ovarian drilling is to eliminate many of the follicles and cells that are producing extra androgens. The procedure is done by *laparoscopy,* which requires general anesthesia and two or three small keyhole incisions in the abdomen. Although the drilling technique sacrifices some healthy eggs and follicles, the presumption is that other follicles and eggs will be given a better chance to develop. However, ovarian drilling does nothing to alter a bad metabolic environment of overnourishment and insulin overproduction.

We will never know for sure which factors eventually eased Lesa's Syndrome O problems of ovarian confusion and ovulation disruption. It is possible that ovarian drilling helped reduce androgen production in Lesa's ovaries, thus allowing a follicle to eventually develop when fertility drugs were used. Of course, Lesa was simultaneously working hard with a personal strategic nutrition and exercise plan. She lost over fifty pounds and felt that her metabolism, insulin, and diabetes were under the best control of her life. If pregnancy was to be in the cards for Lesa, she knew that diabetes and obesity was a disastrous combination. She notes: "I think my ovaries were very resistant at that time because my body was still healing from the years of abuse. It took years to get my ovaries in the polycystic, enlarged state they were in. The problem wasn't going to go away overnight. I really noticed no particular change after the ovarian drilling. In fact, my hormone levels worsened. I remember being devastated that I had gone through that whole procedure only to make matters worse. Dr. Sawin told me that hormone levels often fluctuate and that I shouldn't be discouraged by the test results."

Fortunately for Lesa and Lyle, persistence, good fortune, and prayers prevailed. After a cycle that combined clomiphene with gonadotropin injections, an ultrasound finally revealed a wondrous picture in early 1999—a maturing and growing follicle. Blood hormone levels for estrogen confirmed that Lesa's follicle was getting ready to expel the egg. Now the odds of conception, just 20 percent, were up to Lesa and Lyle. Two weeks later they learned that they were actually a fertile couple after all. Hannah was born full term and healthy later that year. Lesa credits her ongoing preconception life-management plan as vital to her pregnancy success.

How far-reaching can the SOS Strategies be for restoring health and fertility? If the ovaries are a trustworthy guide, it may be possible to completely reverse ovarian confusion and ovulation disruption. Lesa's third child, Daniel, is a testimonial to that assertion. As Hannah and Elizabeth grew a little older, Lesa started to have some new maternal yearnings. She had also been very diligent in her own personal SOS Strategies and was beginning to wonder if her ovaries could work properly. Dr. Sawin performed an ultrasound and found that Lesa's ovaries appeared smaller and less cystic. Lesa was taking birth control pills at the time, which can temporarily shrink the appearance of polycystic ovaries.

In late 2001, Lesa tried an experiment for which I was happy to give advice from nine hundred miles away. She wanted to determine if she was now capable of ovulating on her own, with no fertility pills or insulin-regulating drugs. Lesa stopped taking BCPs. After a few weeks, no period was forthcoming, suggesting that ovulation had not taken place. Lesa's disappointment then turned to surprise as shortly after her first spontaneous menstrual period did finally happen.

No woman on the planet could have been happier to see her own menstrual period. Although I didn't want to dampen Lesa's enthusiasm, I had to tell her that there was no way to know for sure that she had actually ovulated prior to her spontaneous menses. I suggested that she have a progesterone blood level tested the following month. Sure enough, a few weeks later Lesa's progesterone level was over 19, a very robust number indicating with 99 percent certainty that ovulation had occurred. Within a month, Lesa was pregnant again, but this time without using any fertility medications.

Lesa's Passion: Helping Others

Syndrome O is here to stay for Lesa Childers. Her inherited tendency to produce and store fat when overnourished will persist for the rest of her life. Although insulin overproduction can be controlled, the diagnosis of diabetes is nevertheless inescapable. Medical endocrinologists assert that once someone is diagnosed with diabetes, that diagnosis stays forever. The sensitivity of Lesa's ovaries to insulin is also inherited, which means she will always be on guard to watch the regularity of her own menstrual cycles and the cosmetic impact of excess androgens in her bloodstream. However, by having this information, Lesa has the free will to accept and control things in her day-to-day life. When asked about her personal ability to gradually heal Syndrome O, Lesa stated that she believes that all women with Syndrome O can benefit from a strategic plan, whether they are interested in fertility or not. "Prevention is the best medicine," she states. "Getting control of insulin levels means preserving fertility for the future. It also means lowering risks of longer-term health consequences such as diabetes and heart disease."

Lesa believes that her day-to-day challenges with Syndrome O have actually made her a better person, both at home and in her profession as a social worker. "It wasn't easy transforming my life, but it is the best decision I ever made. I wouldn't trade my life now for anything. I am happier and healthier. I live each moment as if it were my most important. I want my life to count for something in this world. Helping other women with Syndrome O is my mission and if I were to disappear today, I think I already have made a difference. That is what matters."

Motherhood brings new challenges to all women. "Suddenly we find ourselves with a little human being who needs us for almost everything," states Lesa. "As they grow, new challenges to our own health arise. Women with Syndrome O must remain healthy to enjoy all the blessings of motherhood, and even grandmotherhood! Let us also not forget we are setting examples for our children. If they see us eating right and exercising, chances are they will value that behavior also. Strap that baby into a Snugli and head off for that walk. Get outside and play with your children; run, jump and turn flips. Invite older children to join you in exercise sessions. Make them a part of the plan."

Lesa's commitment to helping others has manifested itself in several ways. When I first met Lesa in 1999 she was serving as an active volunteer and regional chapter coordinator for the Polycystic Ovarian Syndrome Association (PCOSA). This premier organization (www.pcosupport.org), founded by Christine Gray DeZarn in 1995, has served thousands of women around the world with up-to-date and reliable information, written and Web-based materials, and resources for peer-based group support. Annual conferences have been an important avenue for women to come together, learn from professionals, and exchange information. Lesa has offered many hours of time to the PCOSA through group leadership, establishment of new chapters, and as invited speaker to conferences throughout the United States.

In 2001, Lesa and I both realized that there was an unmet opportunity to offer the power of positive thinking and strategic action to women with Syndrome O. With some significant brainstorming and leg work, PCOStrategies (www.pcostrategies.org) was conceived as a 501(c)3 federal nonprofit organization. With the mission of implementing the SOS Strategies for motivated women with Syndrome O, major activities of PCOStrategies have included group workshops and individualized one-on-one coaching. An e-magazine called *O Rounds* is sent quarterly to thousands of people.

"I am a believer in organizing and optimizing one's goals and treatment options," states Lesa. "I often find in my coaching sessions that women with Syndrome O have many aspects of their lives spinning out of control—career, school, finances, and relationships—which must affect their overall health. Having a plan to manage these life challenges is an important aspect of each person's specific SOS Strategies."

The SOS Strategies offer something unique—the tools to make change in your life. There is always more to learn about the science of Syndrome O and how women can become empowered to be proactive, rather than reactive. "Nobody at PCOStrategies is a victim," notes Lesa. "We are only victors. That's a very positive message to bring to women with Syndrome O."

Learning From Lesa: Key Motivational Points

Lesa stated once that an unusual friend advised her to form a non-profit organization in order to share her wisdom and enthusiasm with women everywhere. As she meets her daily challenges, which she now views as opportunities, Lesa states that she is happier now than she had ever been. Some key points to consider:

- Lesa has three miracle children who came to her family through vastly different circumstances and experiences. She is a walking journal of family building and perseverance.
- Syndrome O may have started in childhood for Lesa. She ate an abundance of unhealthy foods at an early age and had signs of ovarian confusion and ovulation disruption during puberty and adolescence. Although heredity may be partly to blame, Lesa's family was fertile, productive, and very hard-working.
- In her quest for good information, it took quite a long time for Lesa to be properly evaluated and diagnosed by the medical community. This problem persists currently for millions of women. Today, many opportunities exist for women to get the care and information they need.
- Diabetes affected Lesa at an early age. It provided a significant impetus for her to make changes in her nutrition, activity levels, and overall perspective on life.
- Although needing prolonged and advanced fertility care to achieve her first pregnancy, the Syndrome O Survival (SOS)

Strategies allowed Lesa to be the victor, not the victim. She conceived her second pregnancy spontaneously. Both of her pregnancies were uncomplicated and healthy.

- Lesa's entire life has been dramatically affected by Syndrome O. She now views this as a strong positive force, as she moves ahead to educate, motivate, and stimulate others to change. She is juggling many important activities, including her roles as family woman, social worker, and CEO of PCOStrategies. This should provide inspiration and hope for many other women.

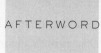

AFTERWORD

Sally, our heroine of the introduction, believed she was a victim of Syndrome O. She is a fictitious person who symbolizes the challenges that millions of other women face with Syndrome O each and every day. Could Sally benefit by careful thought and evaluation of her health and fertility goals? I believe that if Sally keeps an open mind to the strategic concepts of education, motivation, and stimulation, she will gradually reach a higher plane of awareness about her body and her priorities in life. Many women like Sally seek medical consultation to improve their fertility and their health, and they are cautiously optimistic that help is on the way.

As Lesa Childers quickly learned, we all have inner truths, and we must make choices about life activities that are most important to us. The biggest roadblocks to this optimized state are negative thinking and blaming others for our problems. The SOS Strategies encourage women to develop positive thought patterns about themselves, as well as others. It is often necessary, and even encouraged, to lean on others for help and support, especially when making a commitment to major changes in nutrition, physical activity, and management of stressful situations. None of us, neither doctor nor patient, can do it alone.

Do you have personal roadblocks that prevent you from being 100 percent committed to meeting the metabolic and reproductive challenges of Syndrome O? Instead of being frightened away, why not move forward? Women with Syndrome O are blessed with great genes, along with the physical and mental capacity for living each day to the fullest. Armed with determination, confidence, and thousands of "good eggs," I believe that women like Sally and Lesa can survive, thrive, and discover all the terrific things life has to offer. Why can't *you* take control of your life by developing a plan of action? You have much to gain, in wisdom and strength. After all, only *you* can give yourself a fighting chance.

INDEX

ABOUT THE AUTHOR

Ronald F. Feinberg, M.D., Ph.D., is board-certified in reproductive endocrinology and infertility, as well as obstetrics and gynecology, and is the IVF Medical Director for Reproductive Associates of Delaware (www.ivf-de.org). He is an attending physician at the Christiana Care Health System in Newark, Delaware. Dr. Feinberg graduated with honors from La Salle College in Philadelphia and received his medical degree and Ph.D. in biochemistry from the University of Pennsylvania. He completed his residency at Yale–New Haven Hospital and his fellowship at the Hospital of the University of Pennsylvania. Dr. Feinberg served on the full-time faculty of the University of Pennsylvania School of Medicine for ten years, and most recently as adjunct faculty at Yale University School of Medicine. He lectures, consults, and writes frequently about vital women's health issues and research, and has coauthored more than forty articles, reviews, and book chapters. Dr. Feinberg resides in New Jersey, with his wife and three children.